I0791310

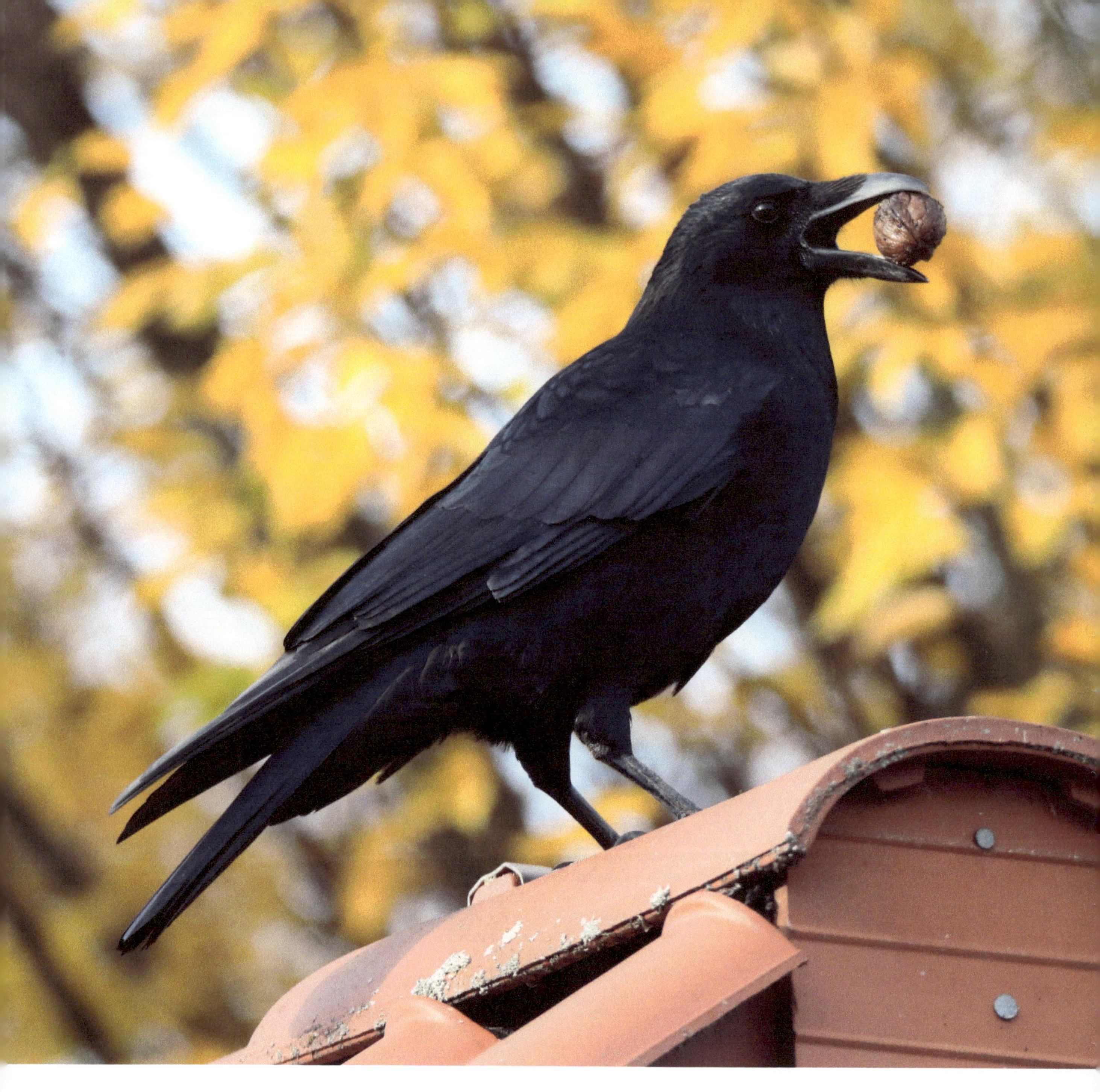

A crow

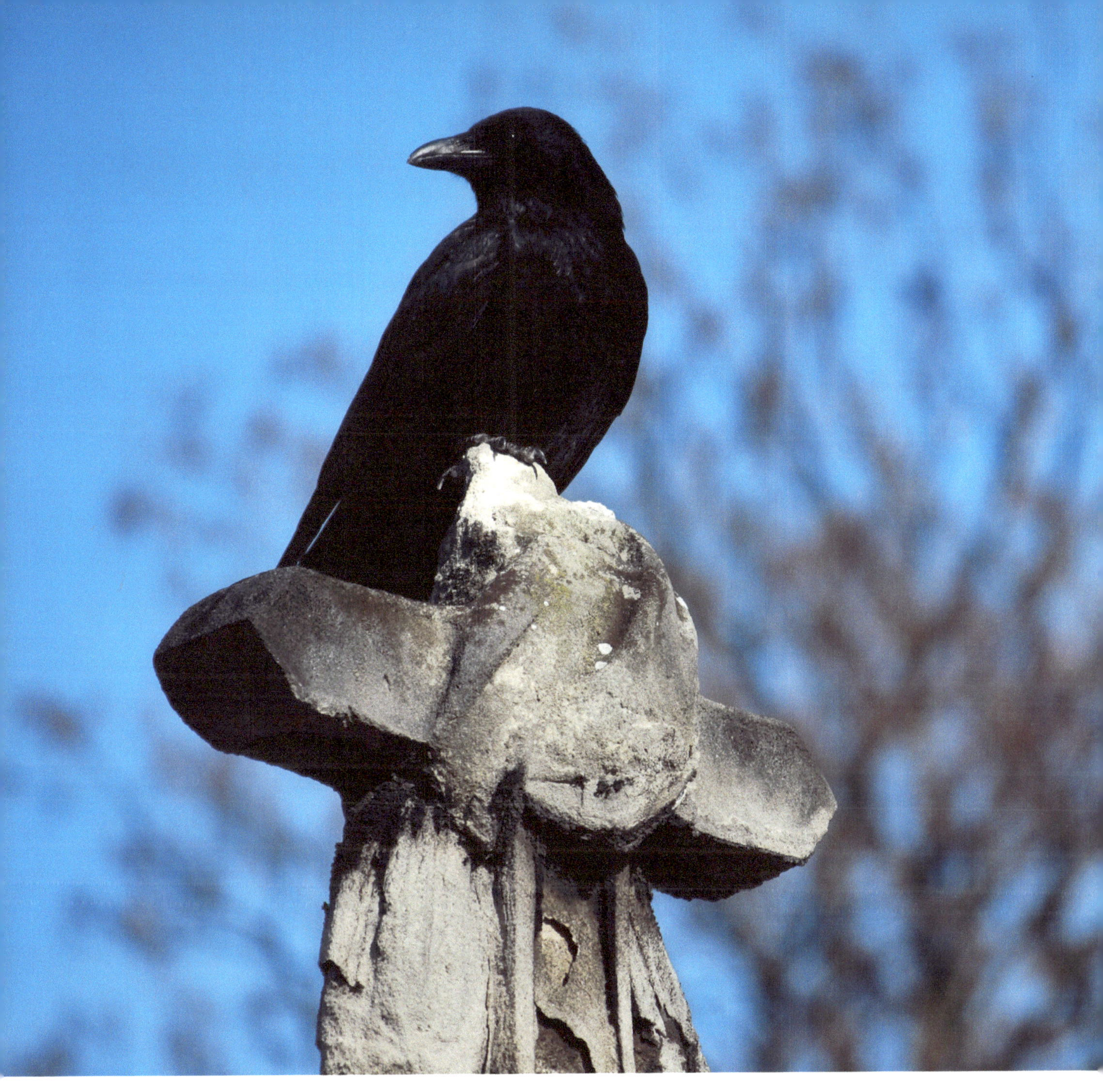

A raven

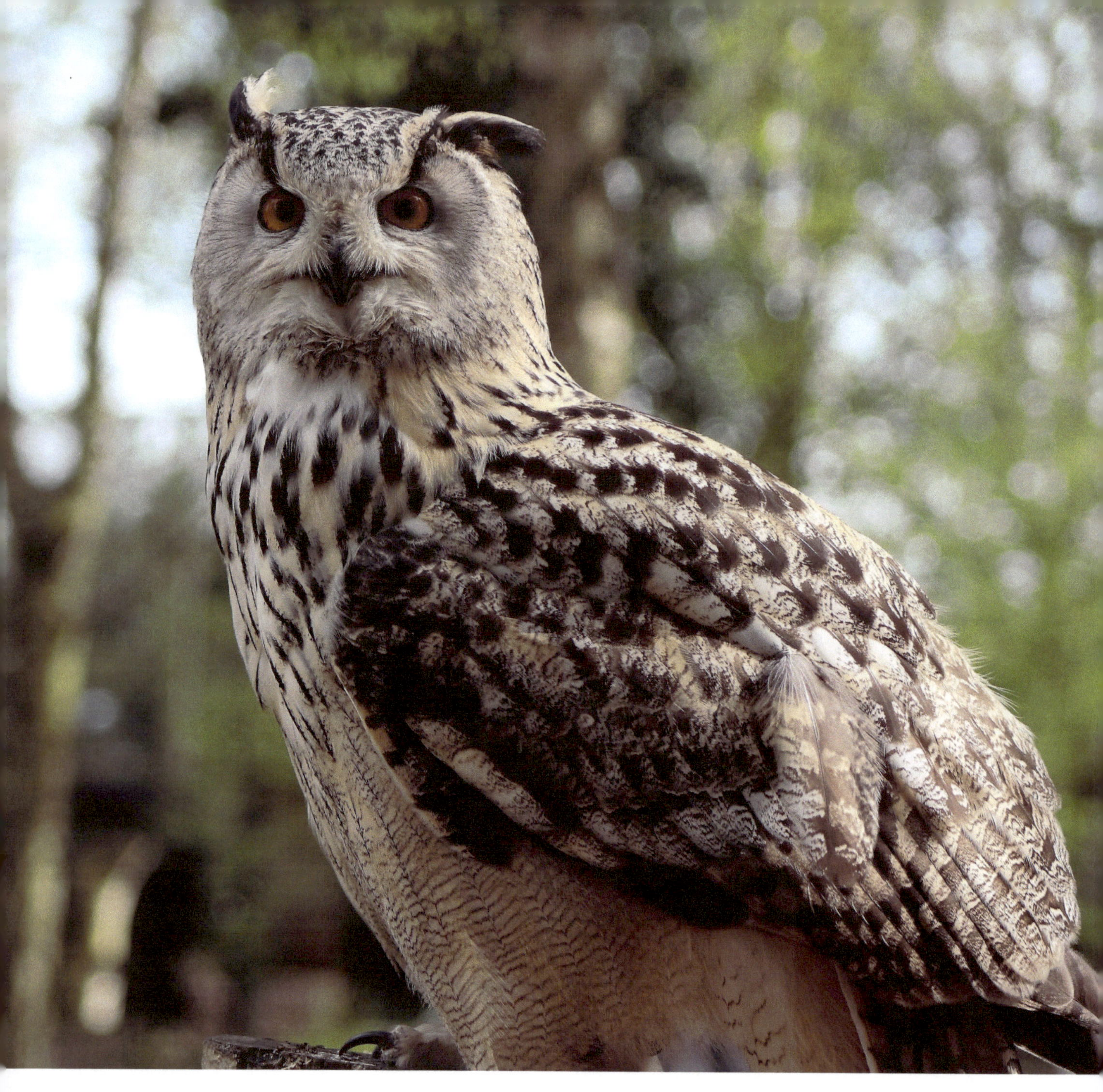

An owl

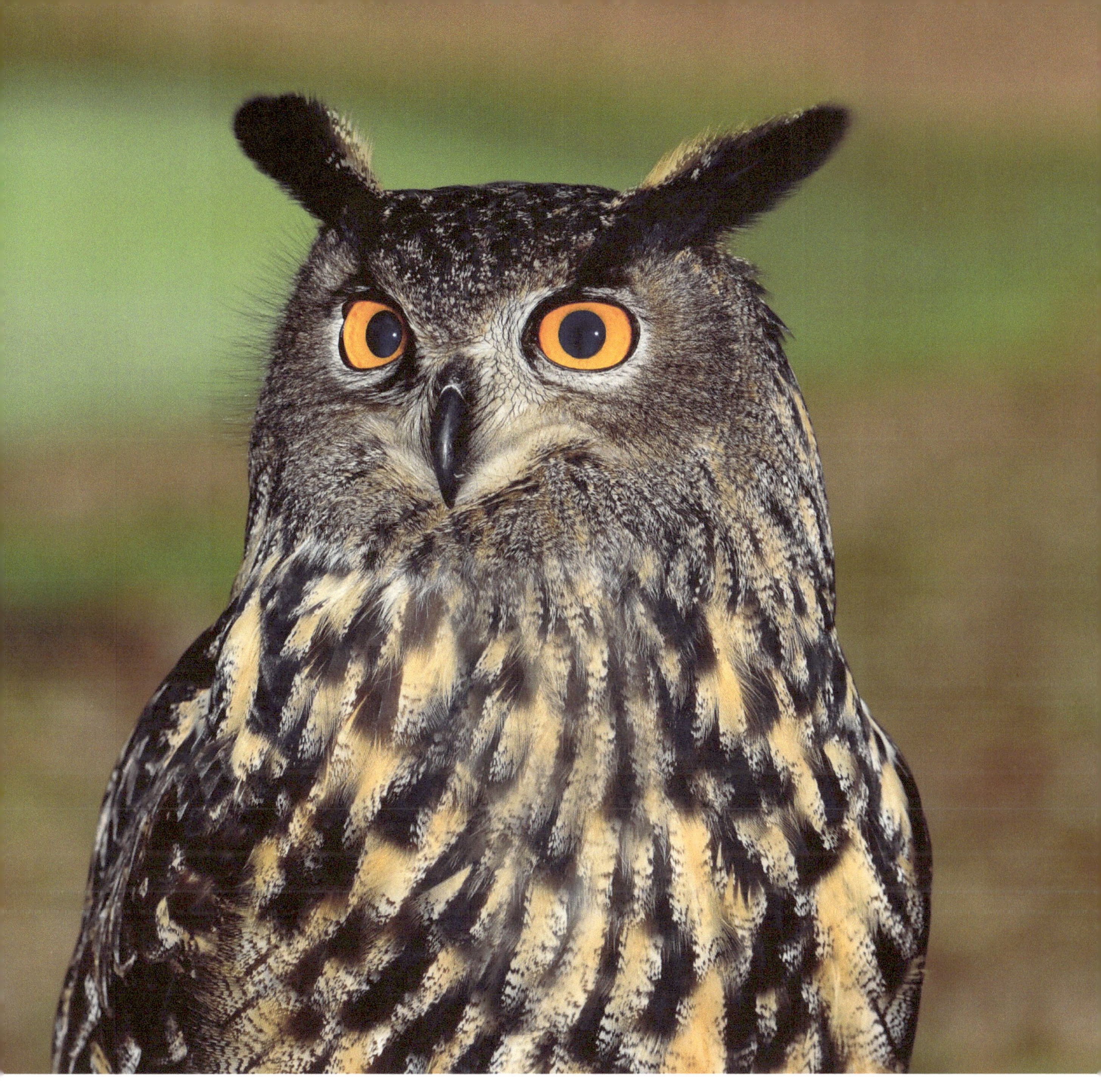

An owl

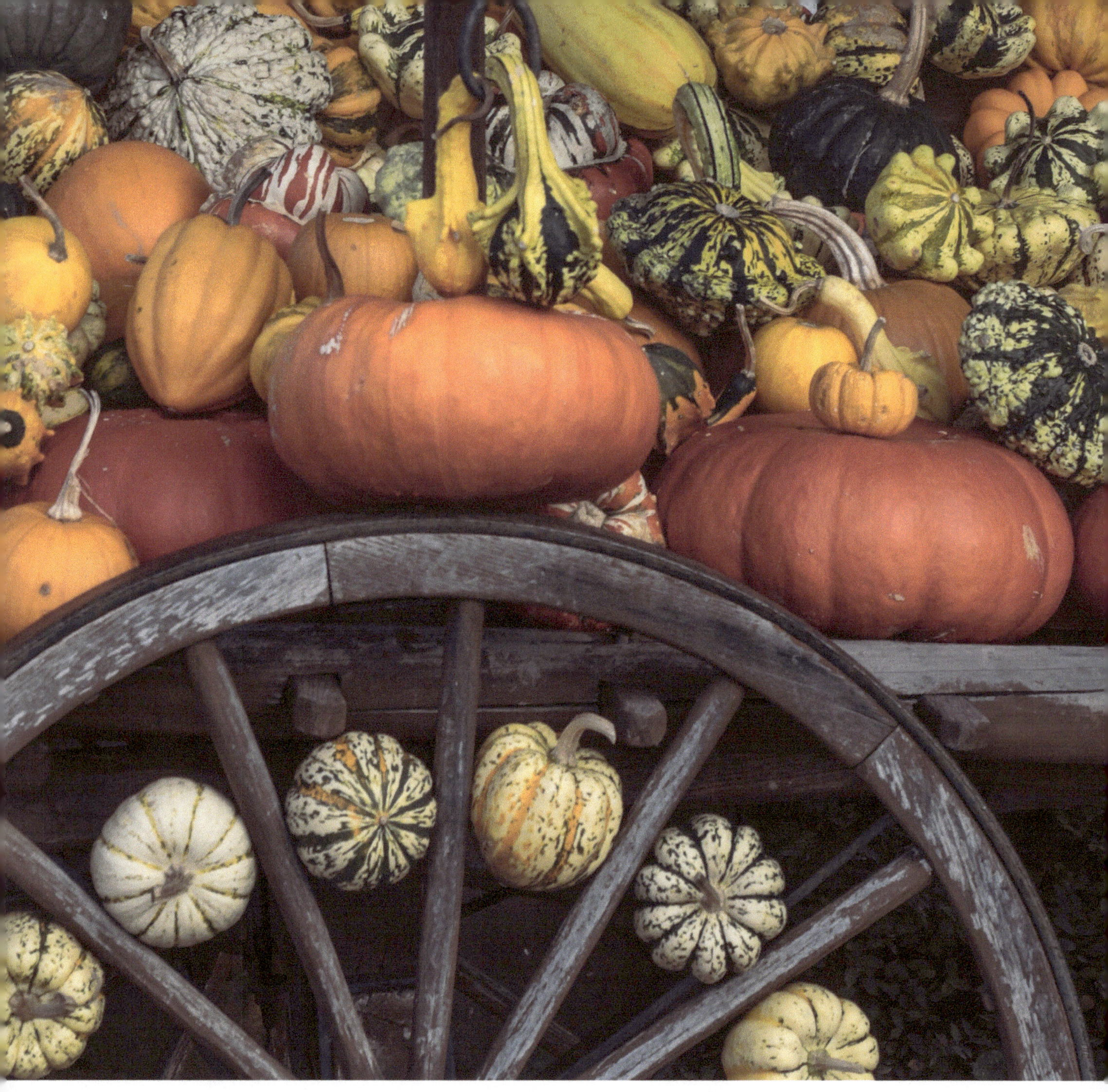

Pumpkins and squashes

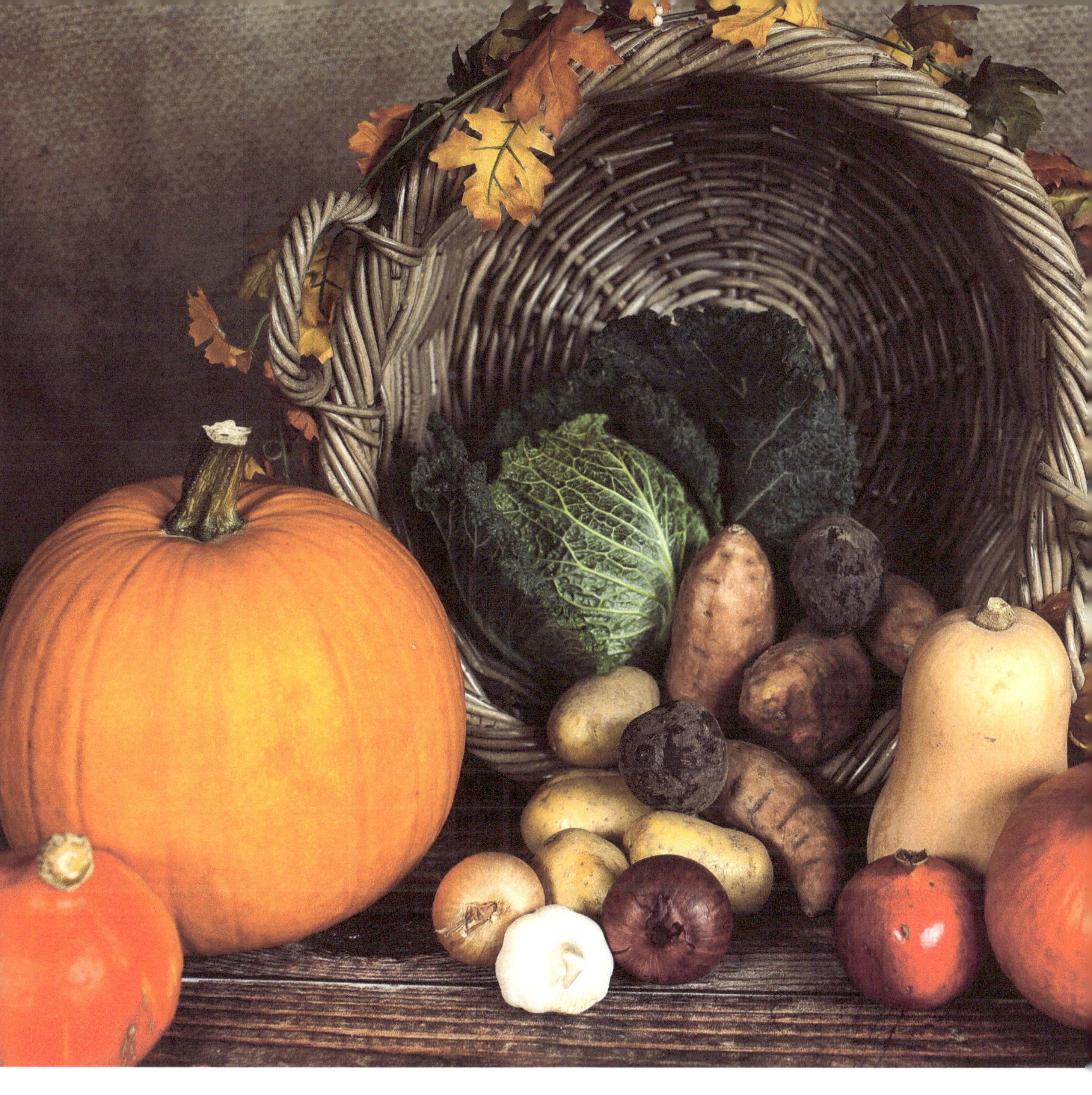

Fruits and vegetables

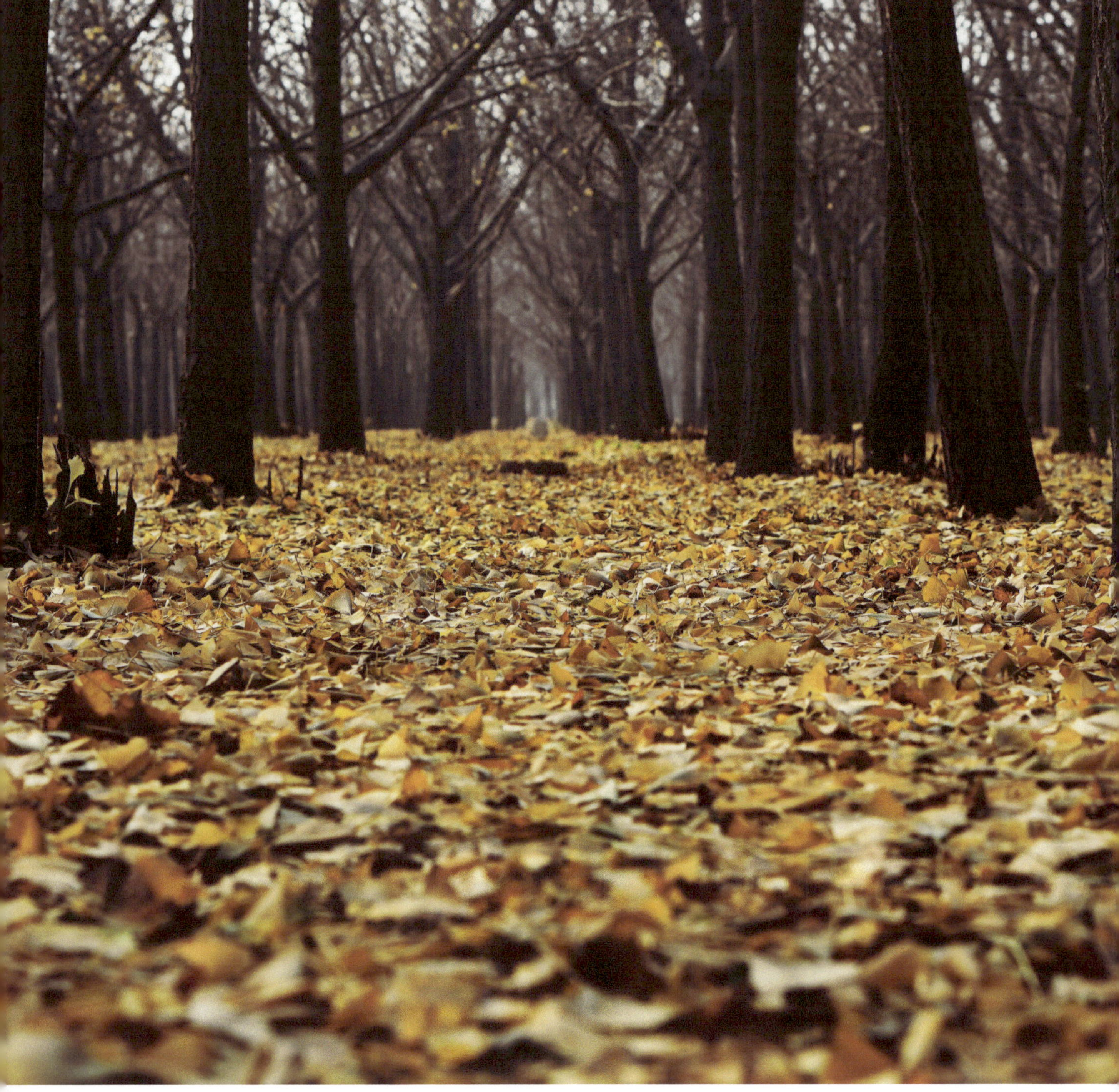

Autumn leaves

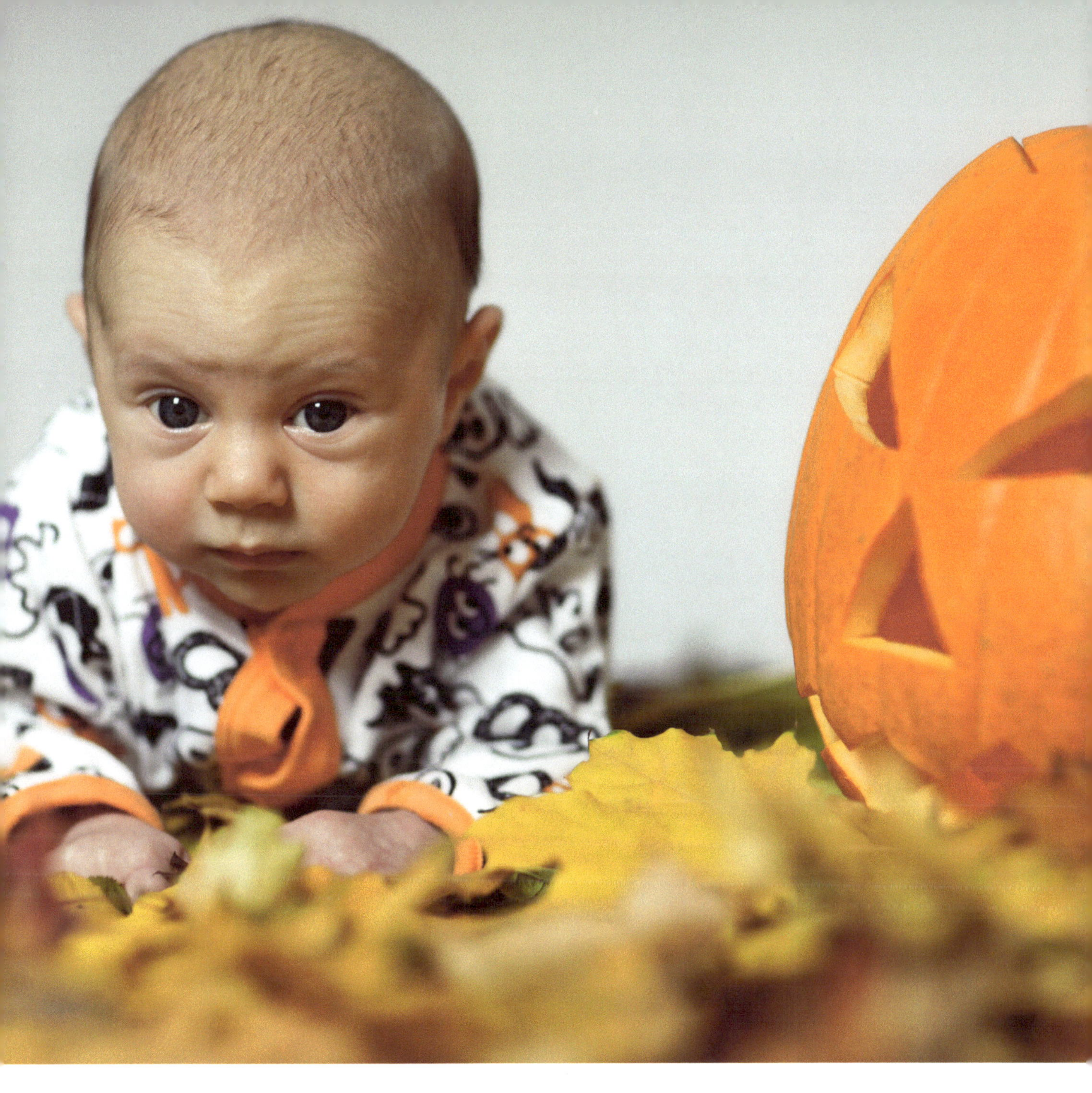

A baby with a pumpkin

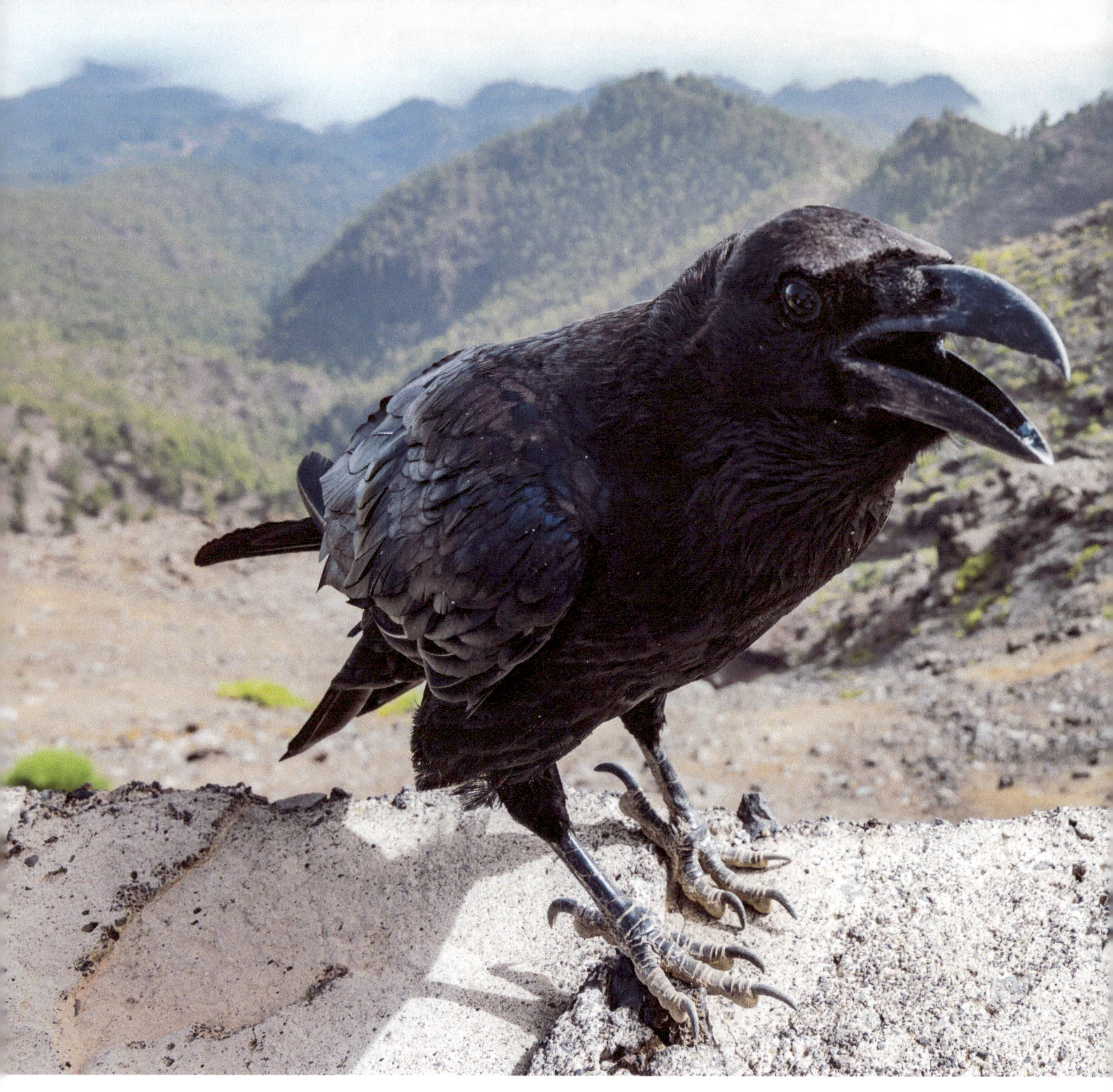

A crow

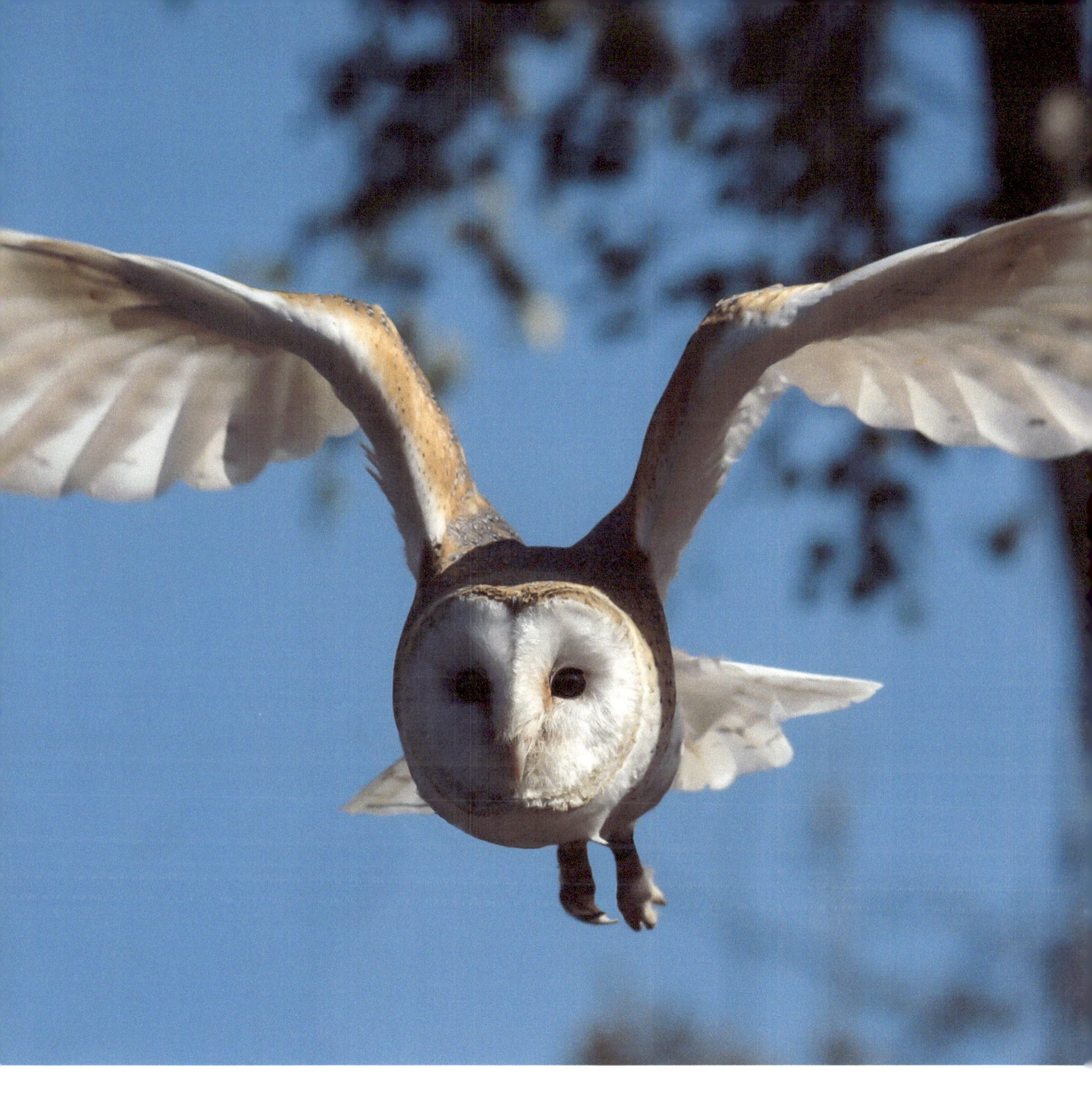

An owl

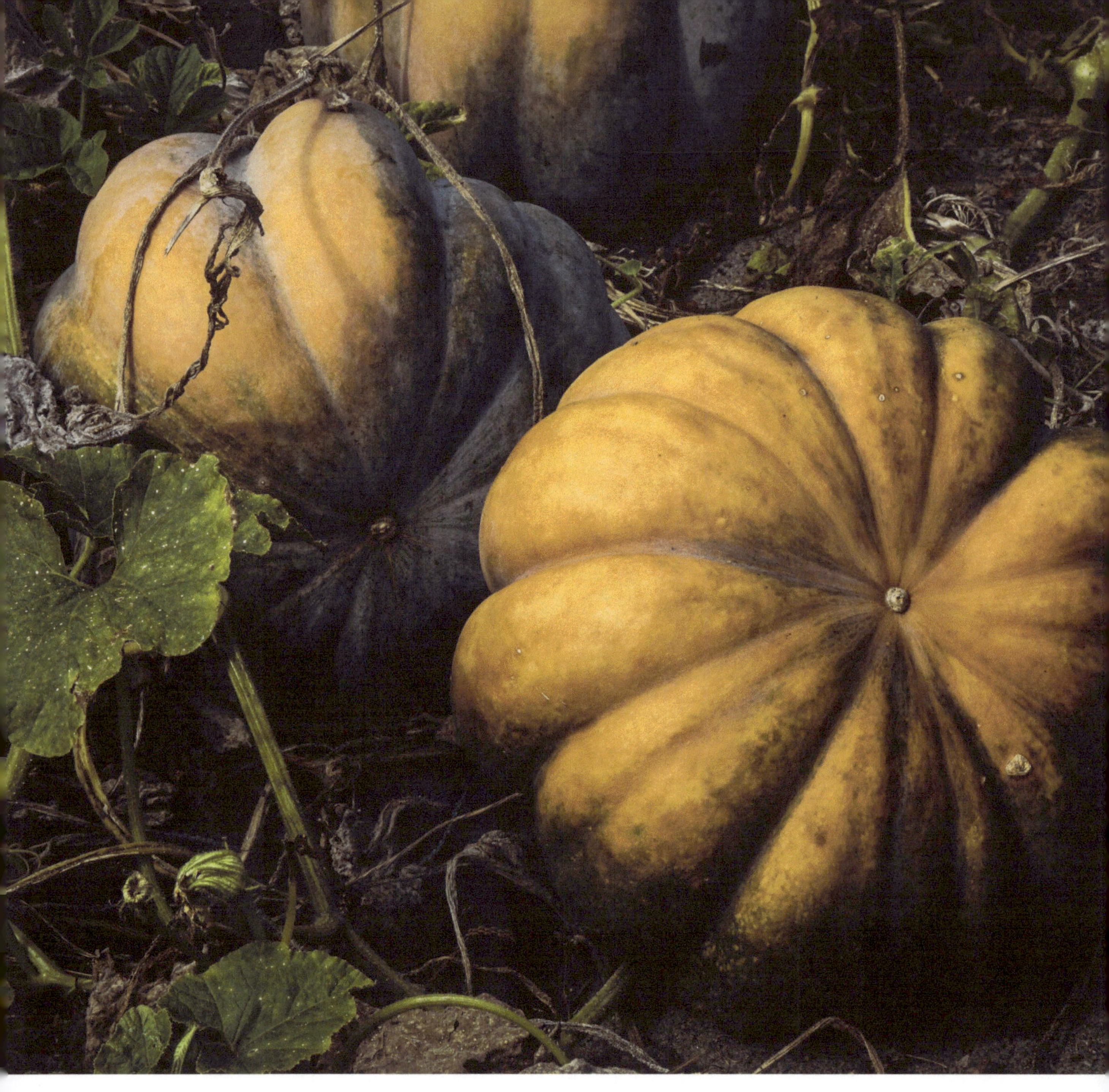

Pumpkins

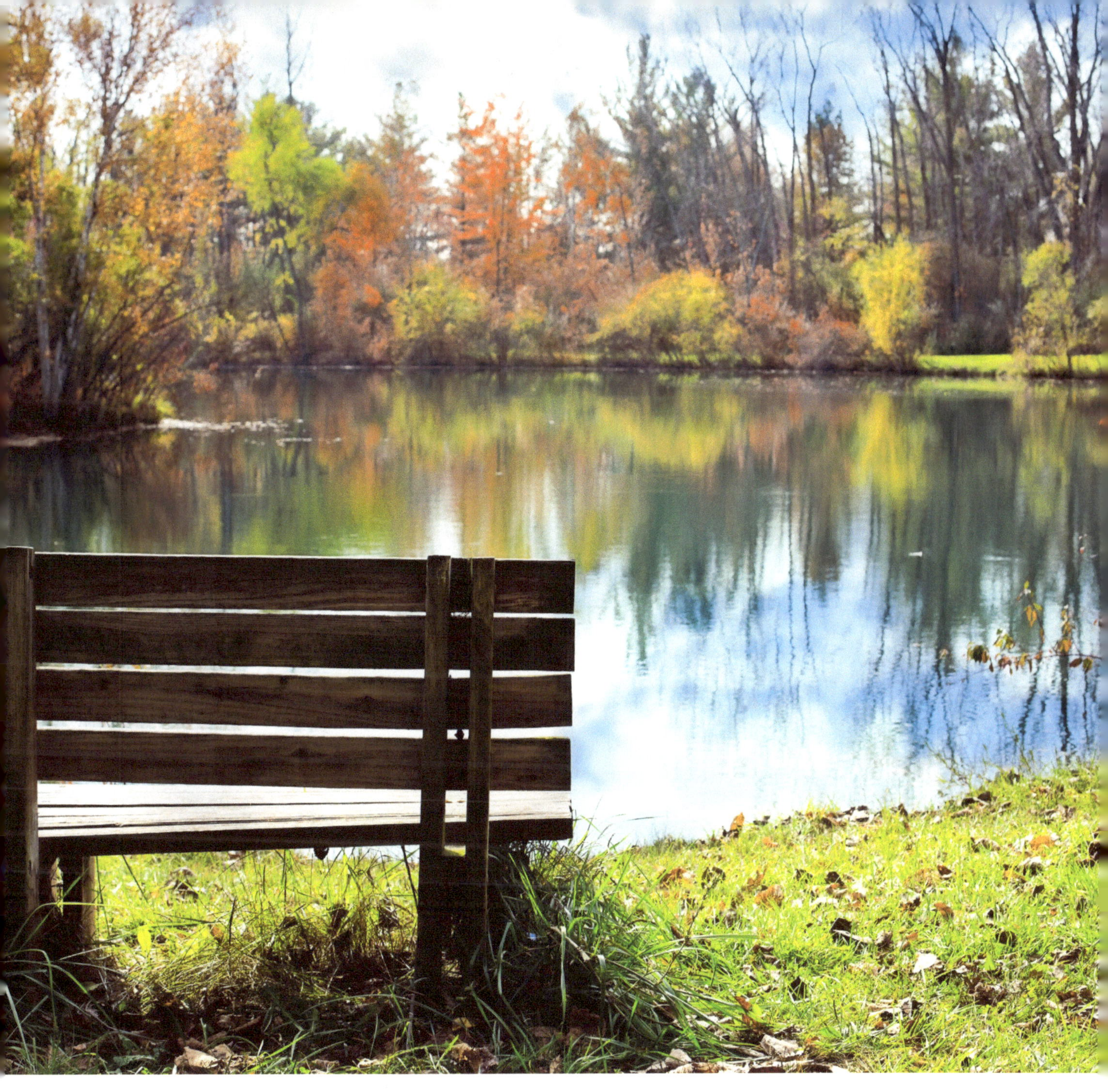

A lake in the fall

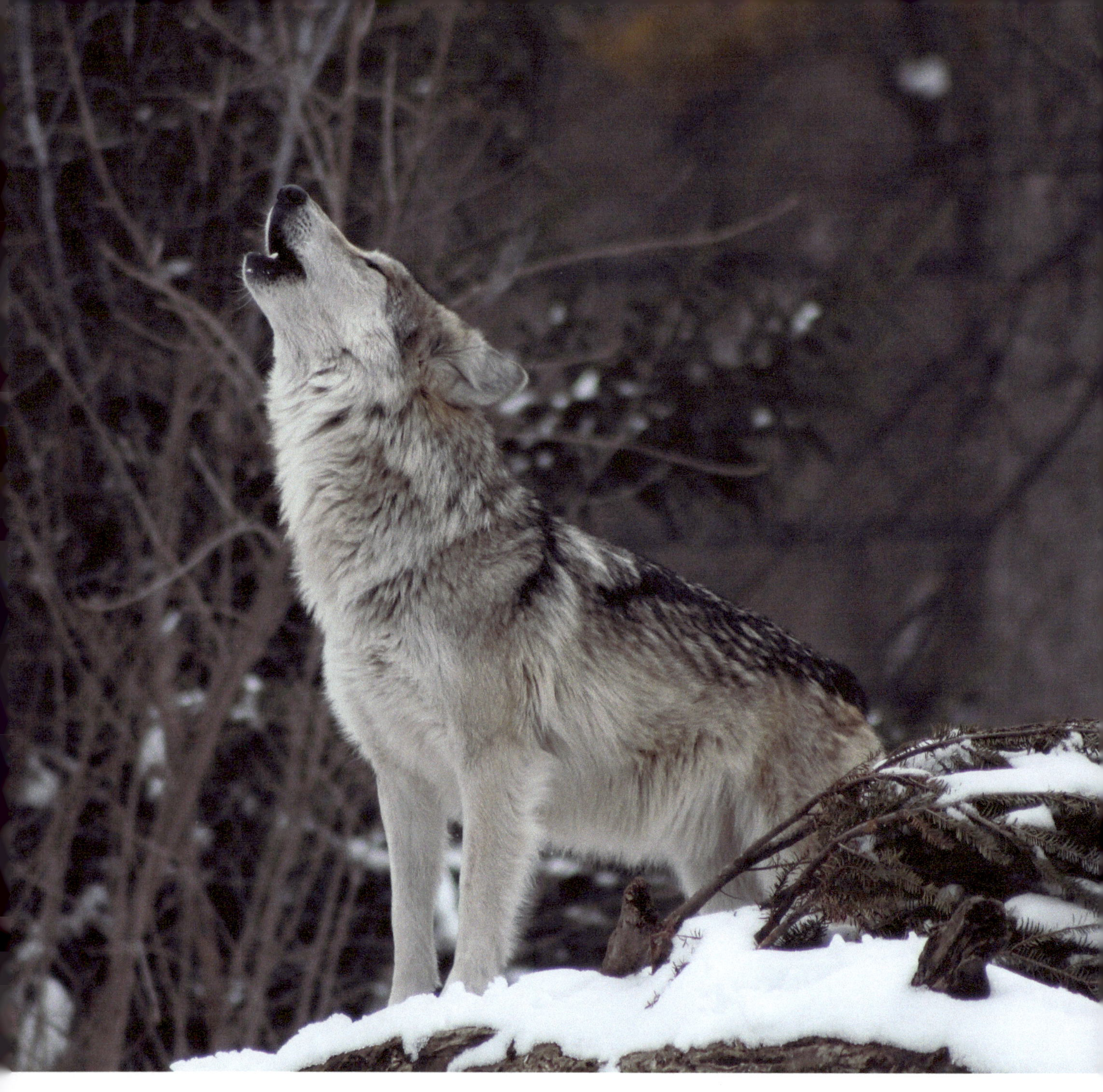

A wolf

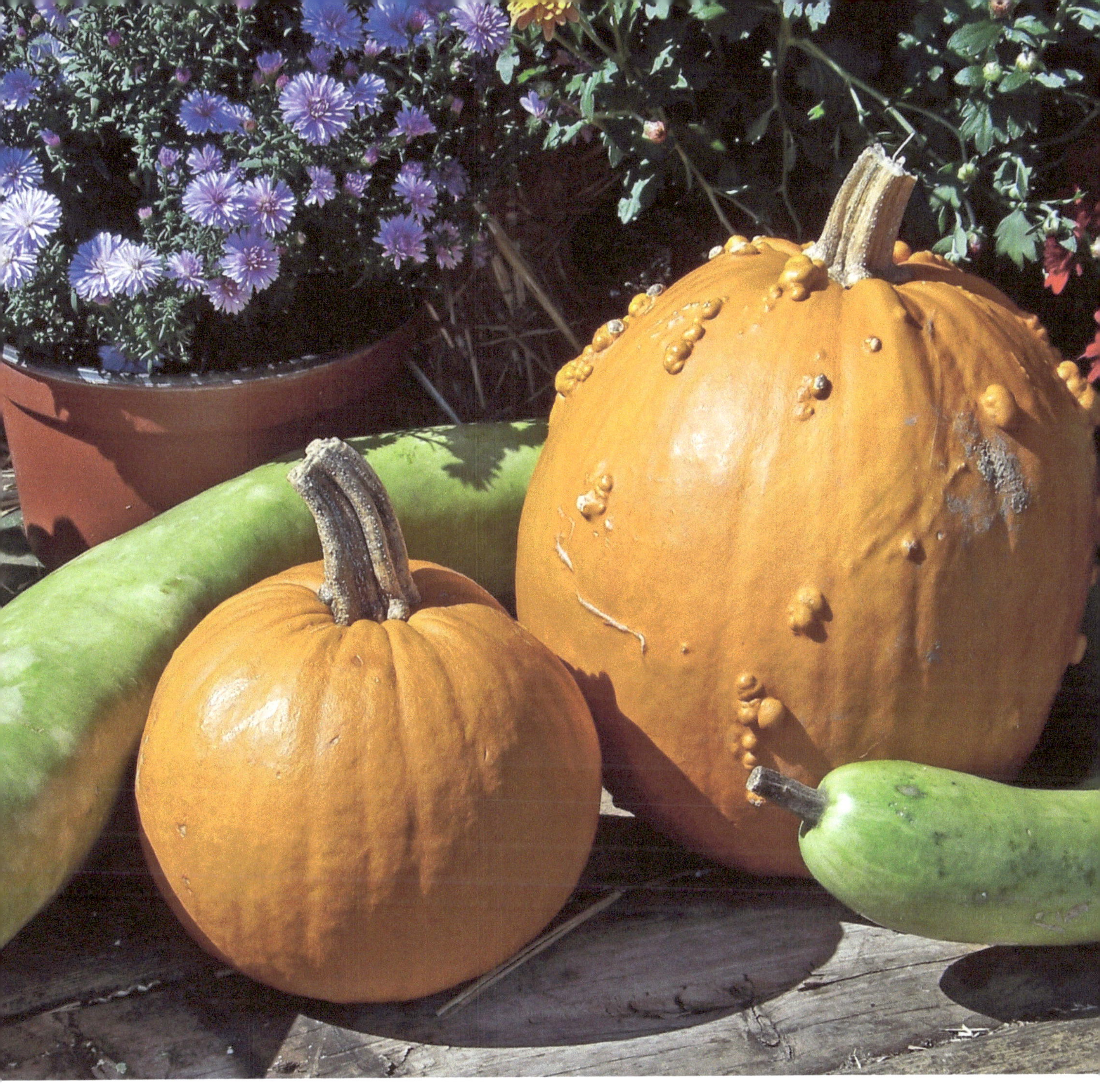

Pumpkins and squashes

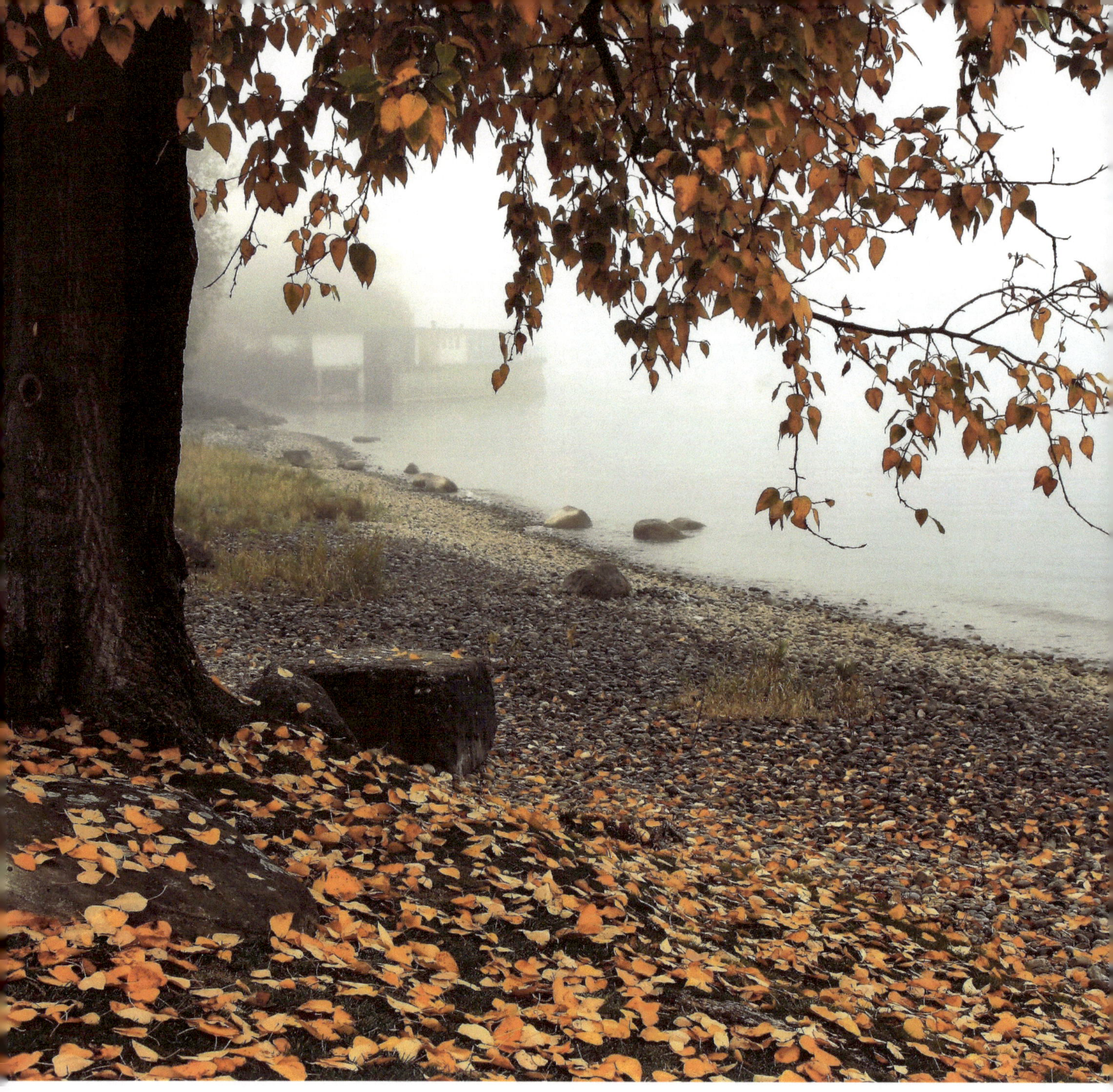

By the lake in the fall

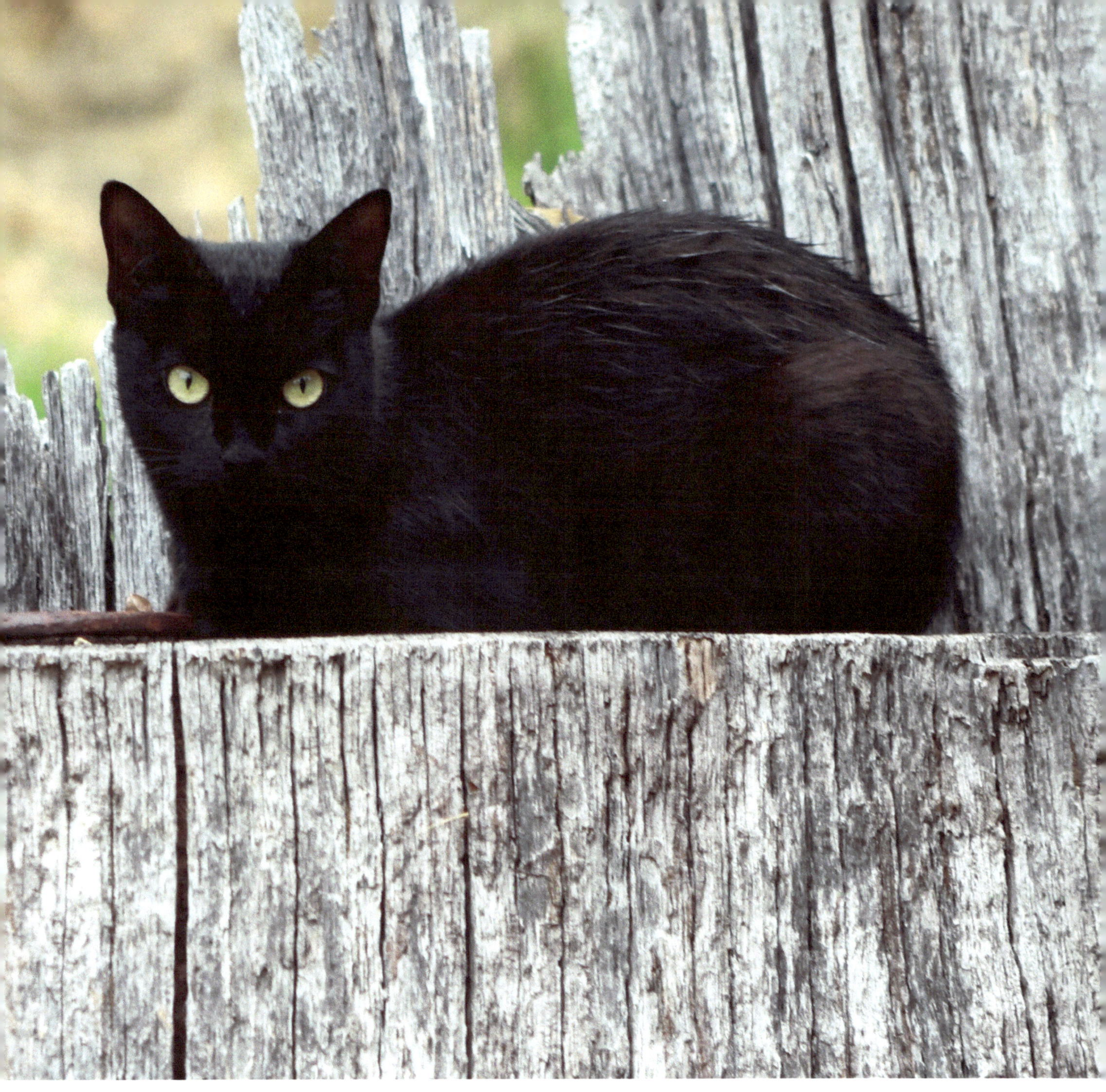

A cat

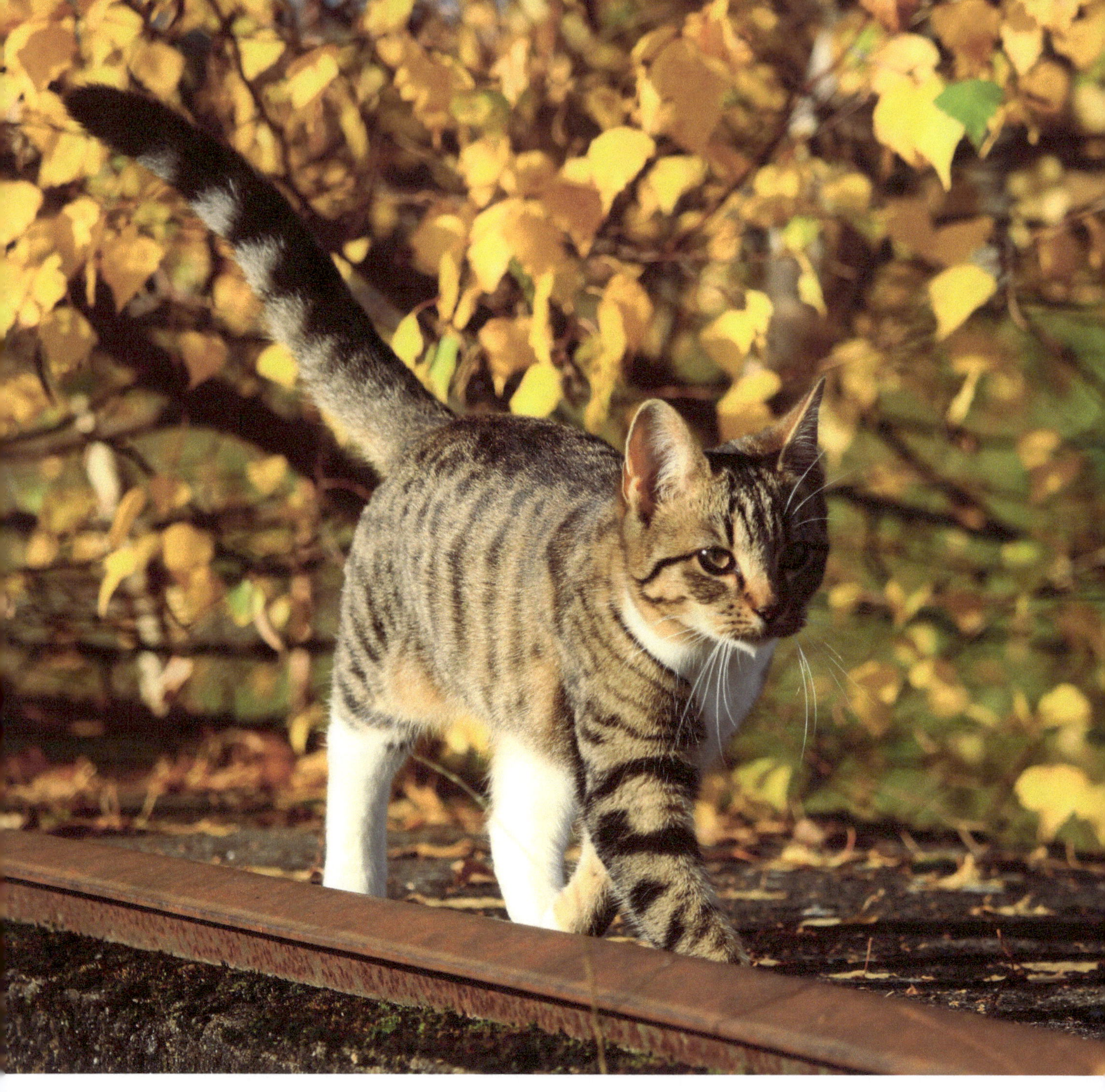

A cat

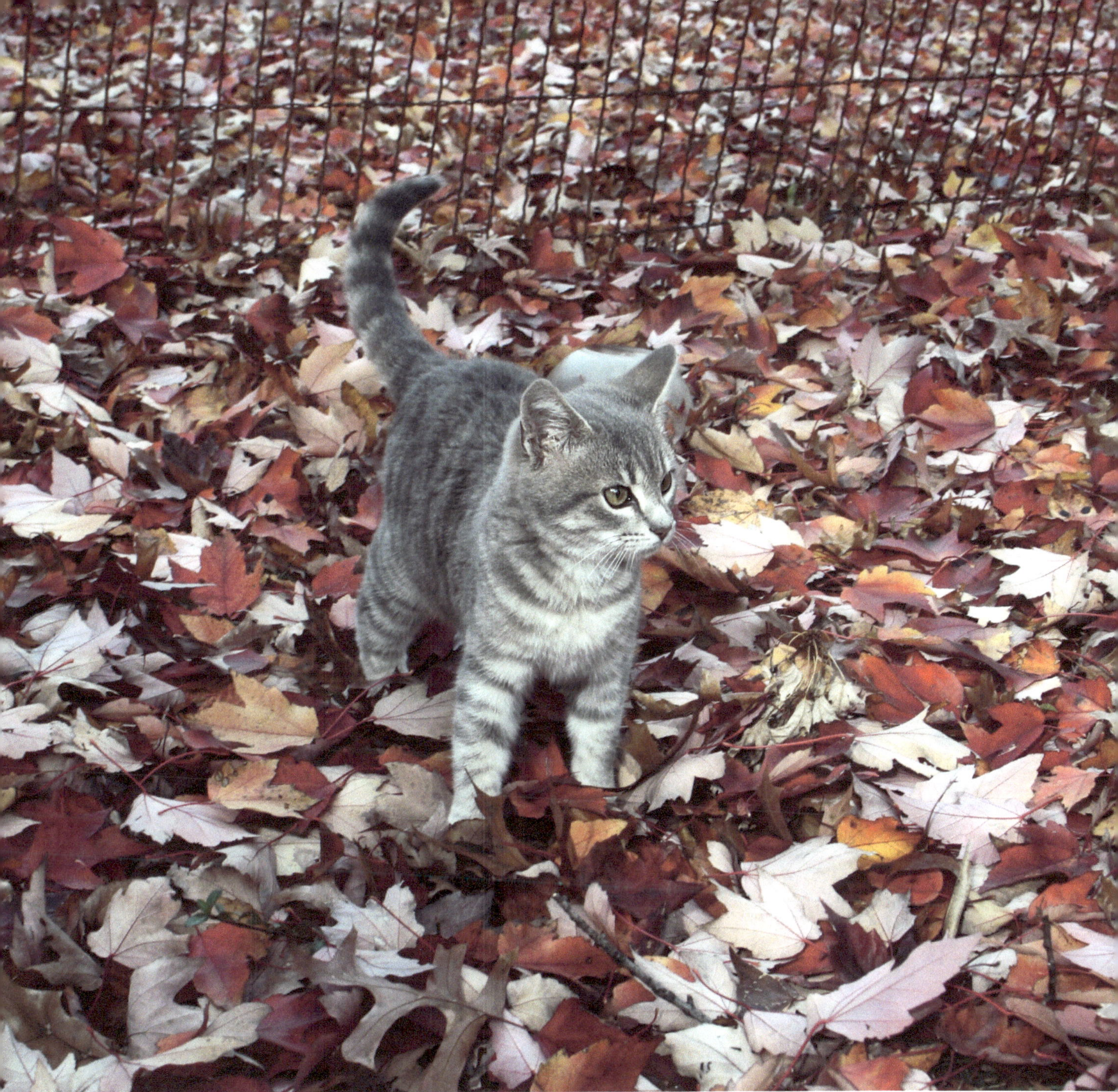

A cat

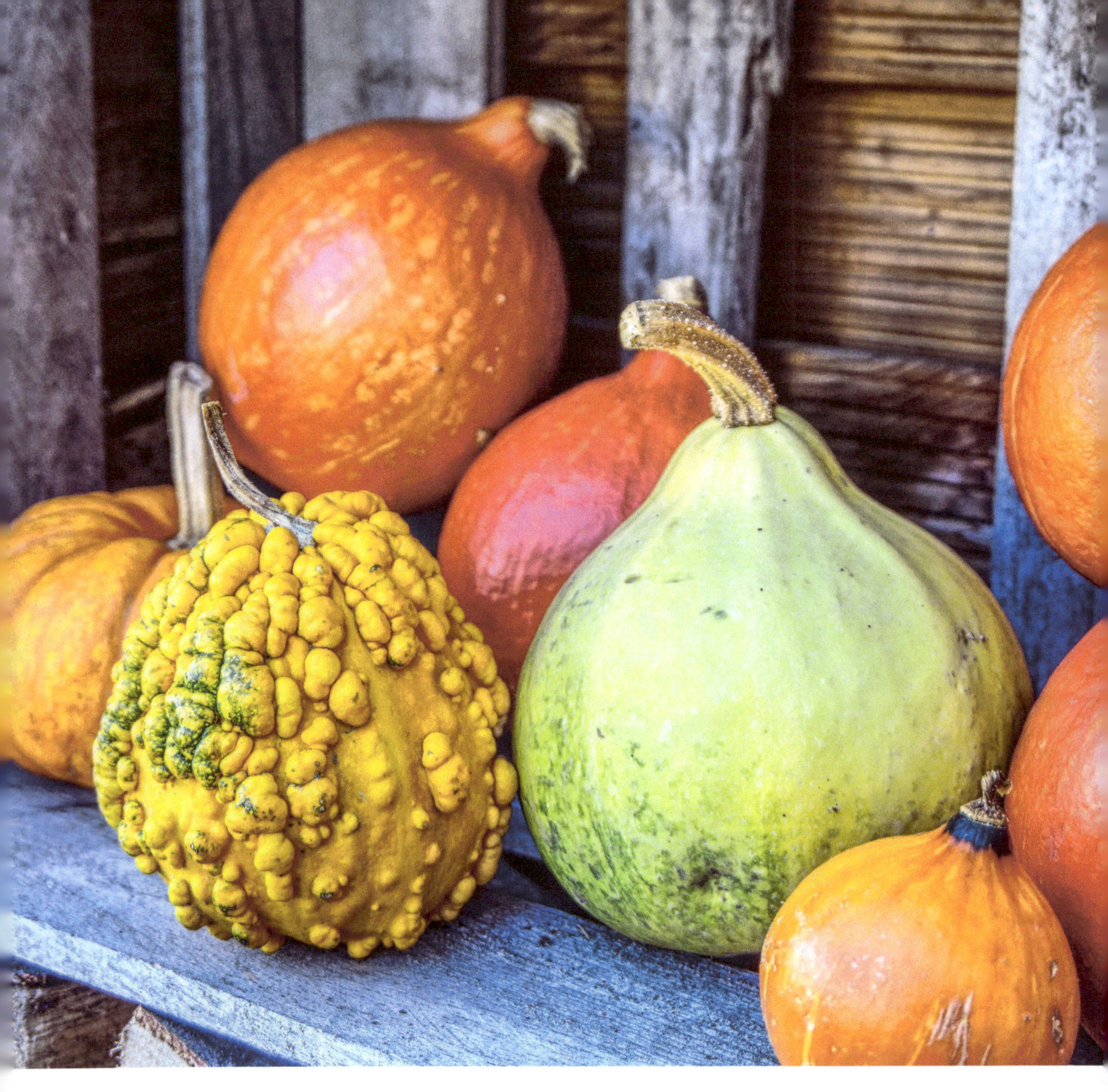

Pumpkins and squashes

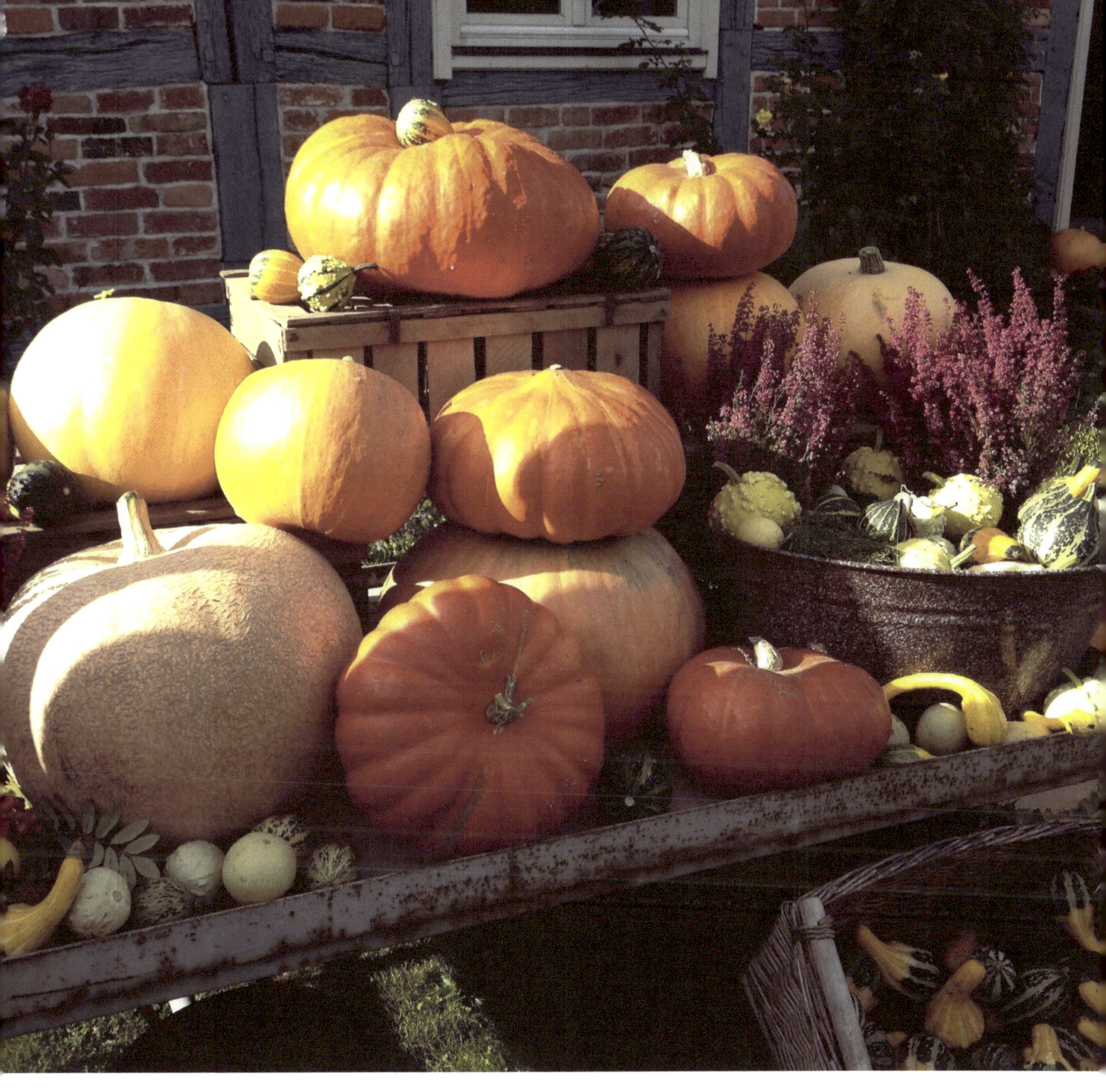

Pumpkins and squashes

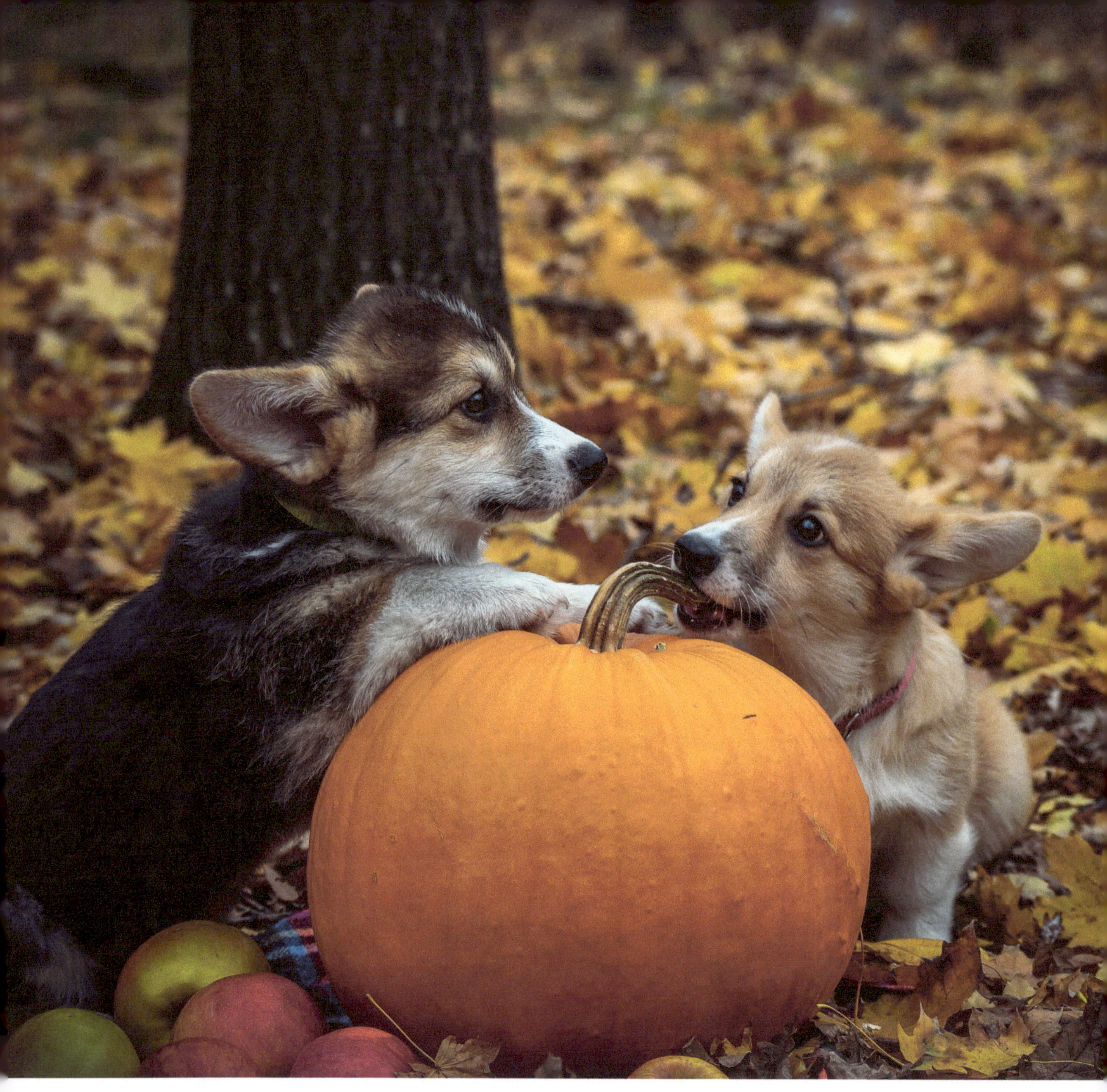

A pumpkin and two dogs

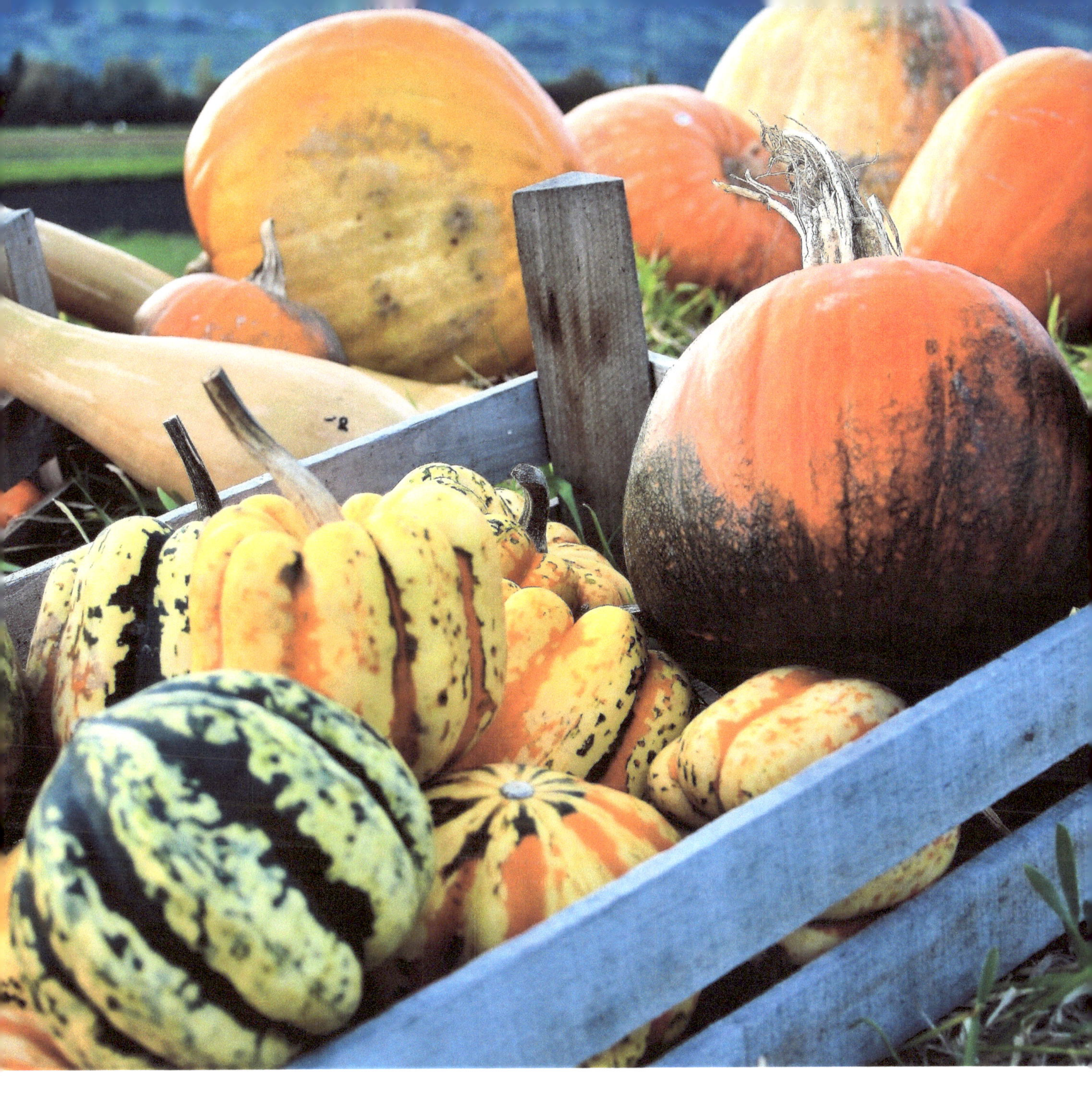

Pumpkins and squashes

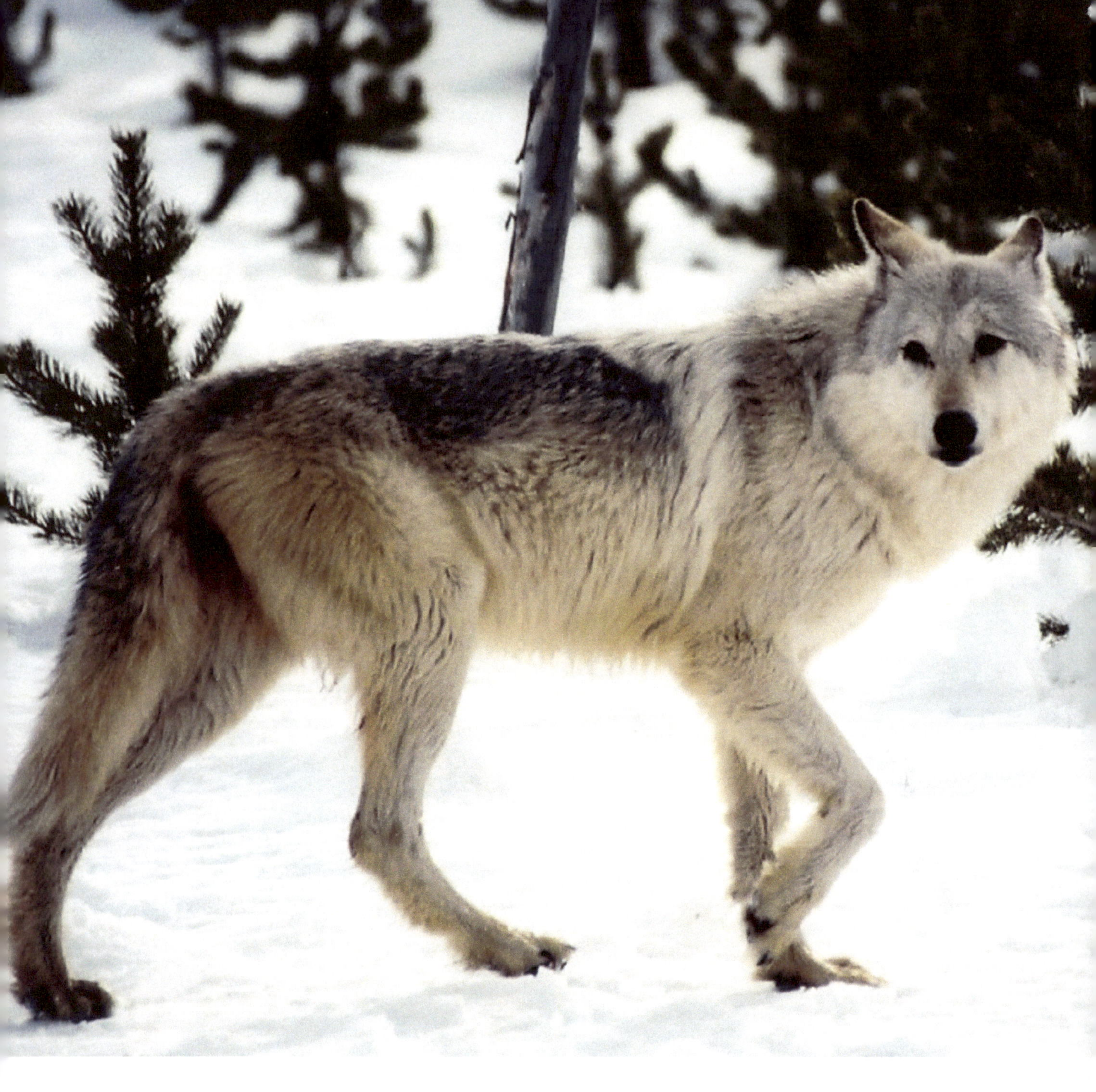

A wolf

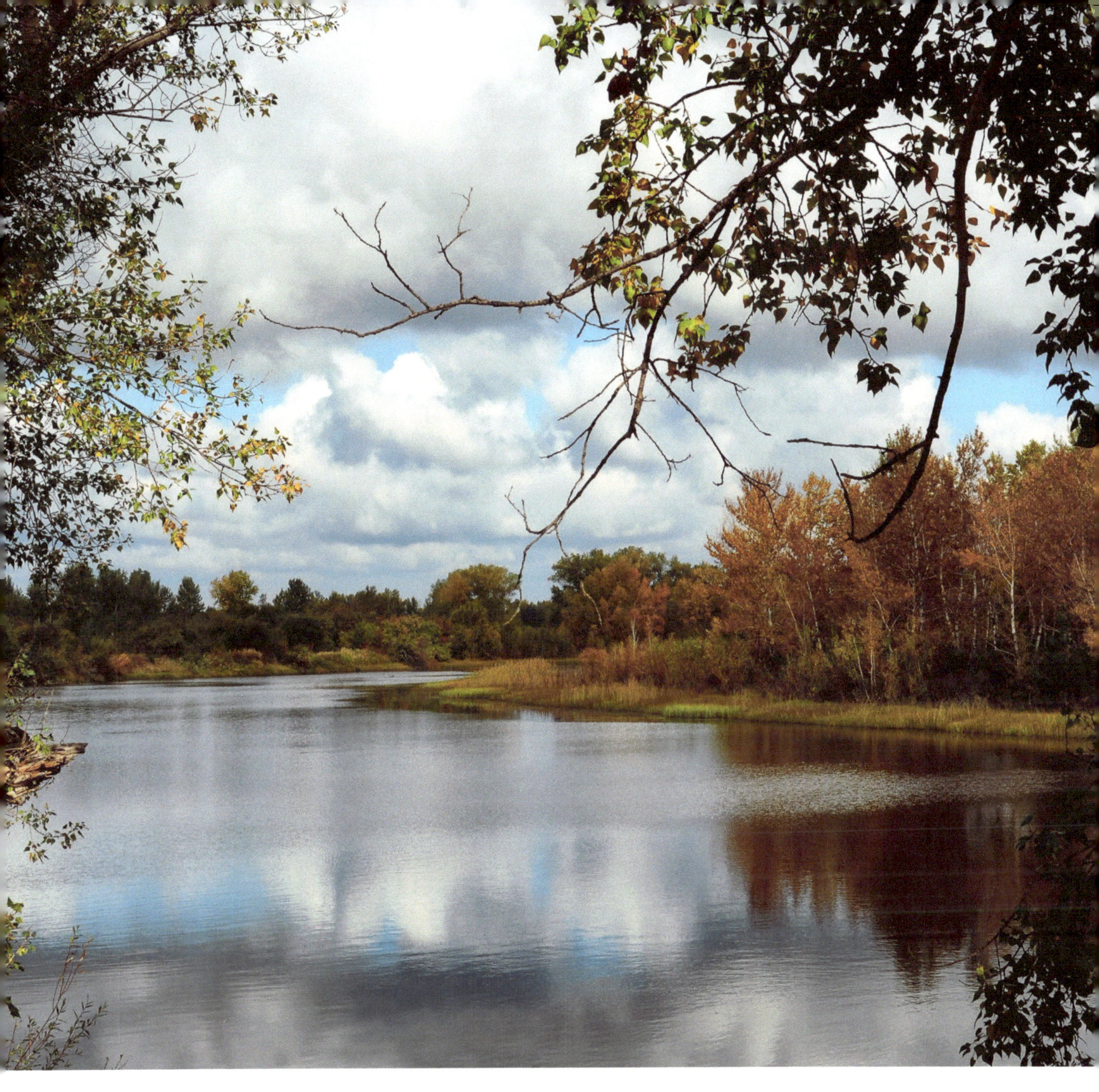

By the lake in the fall

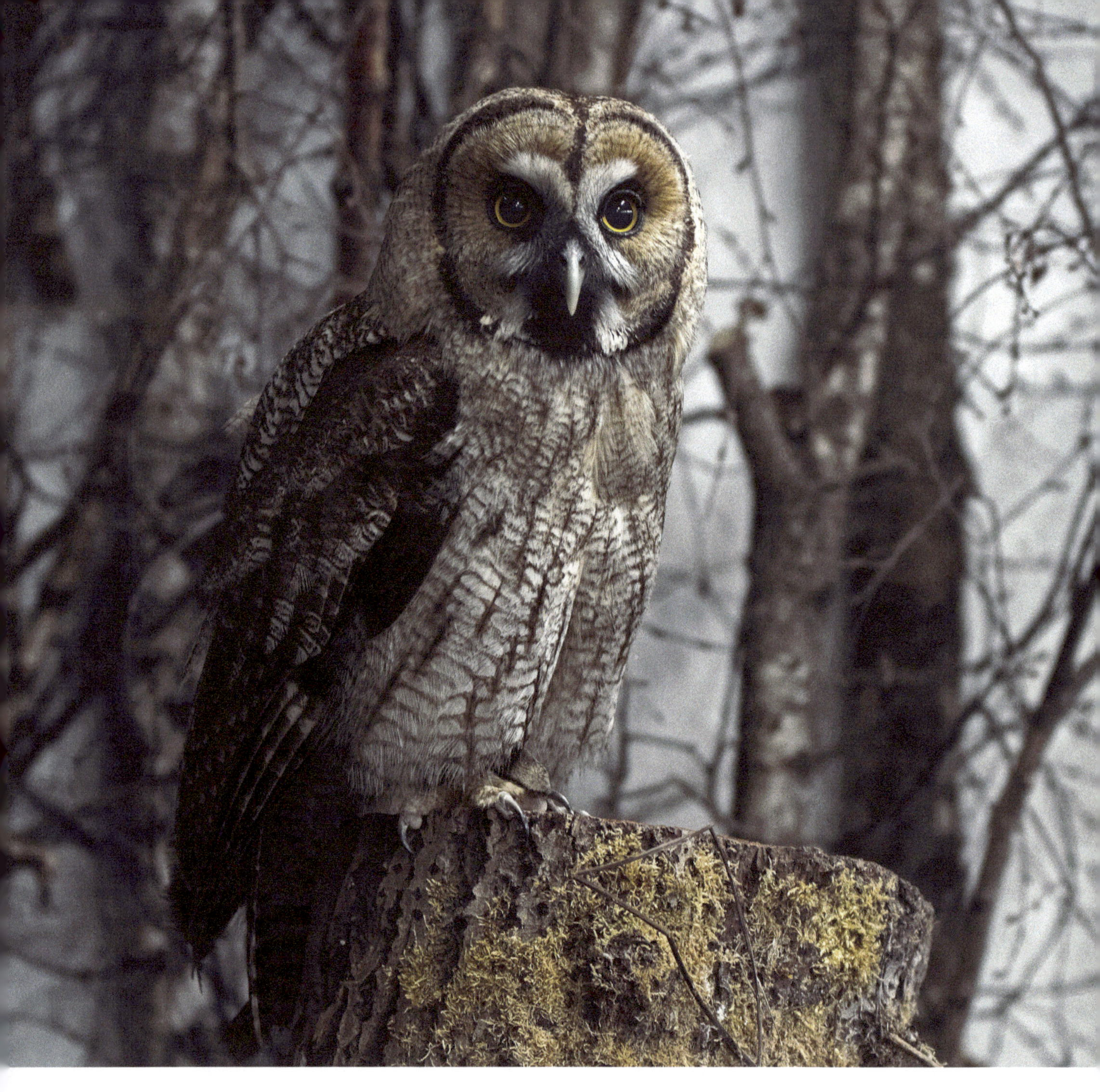

An owl

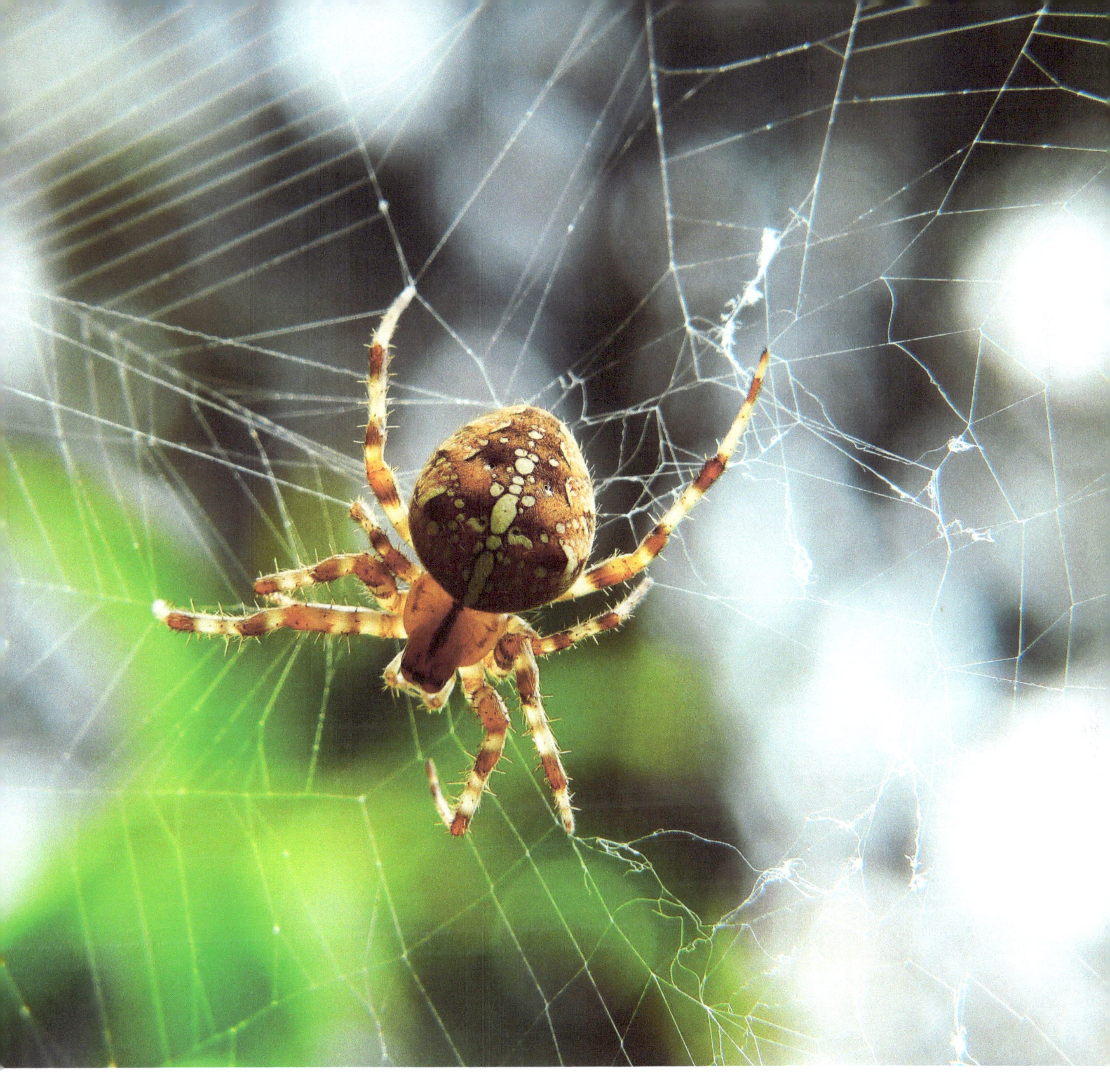

A spider

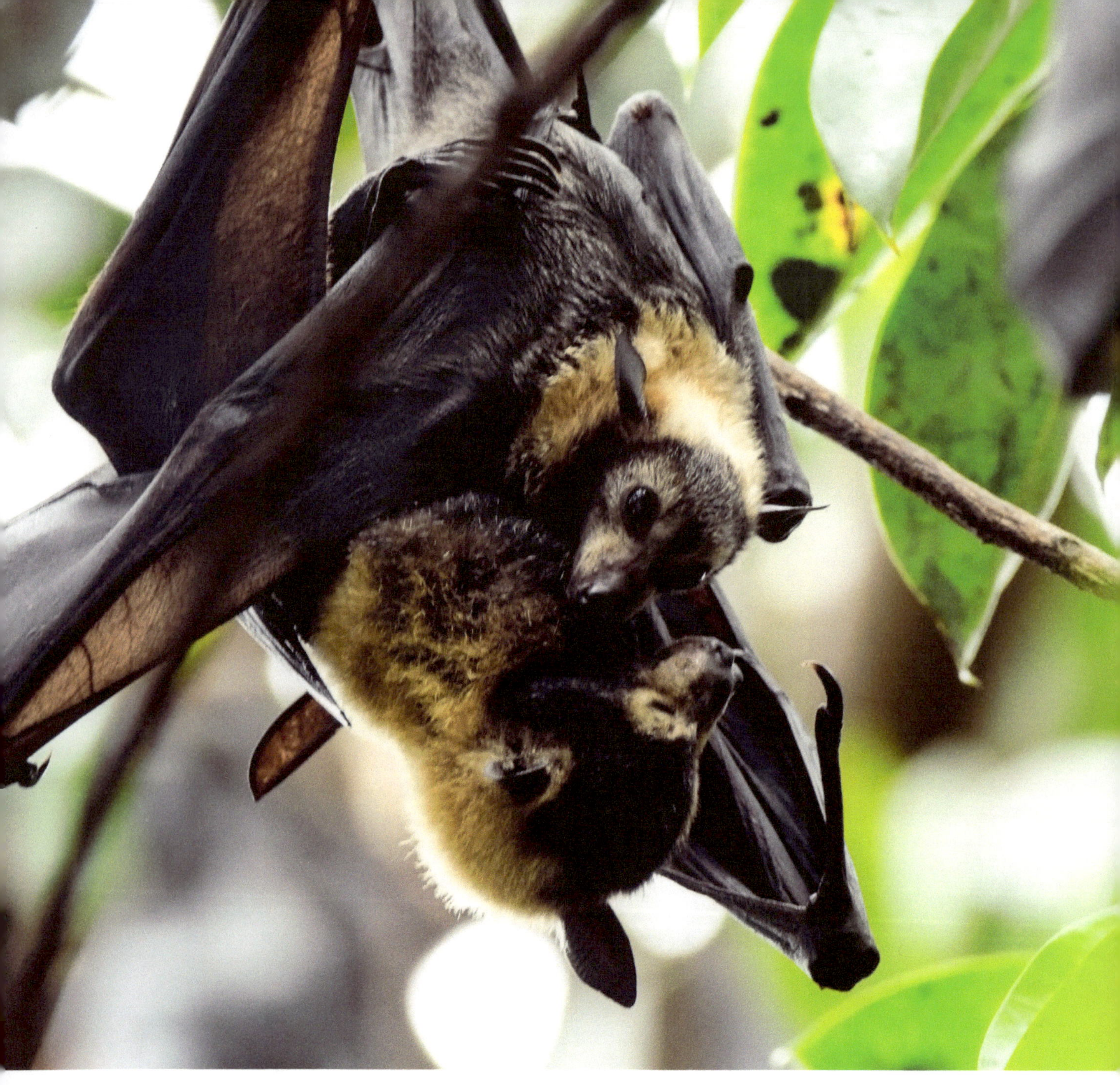

Two bats

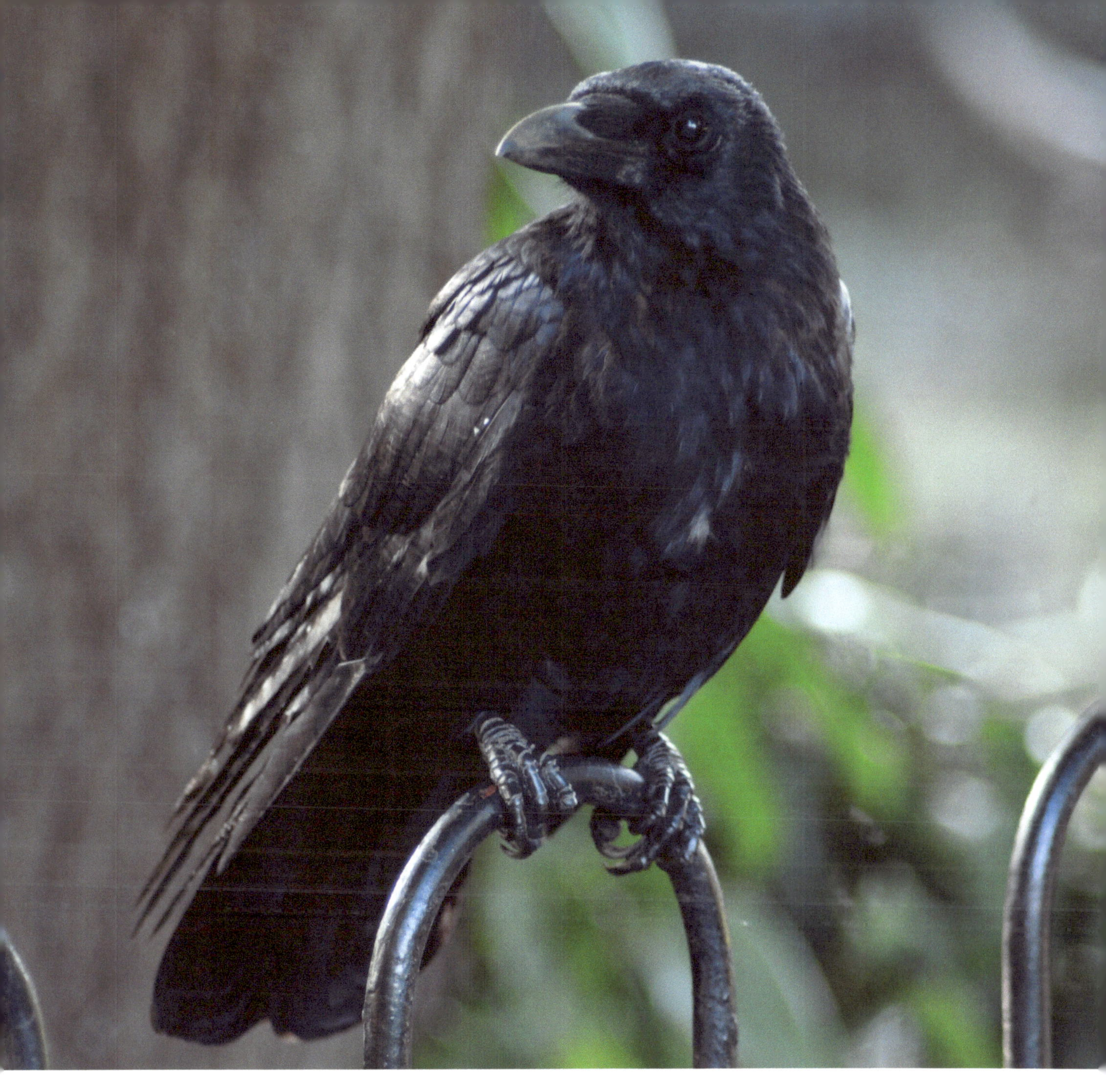

A raven

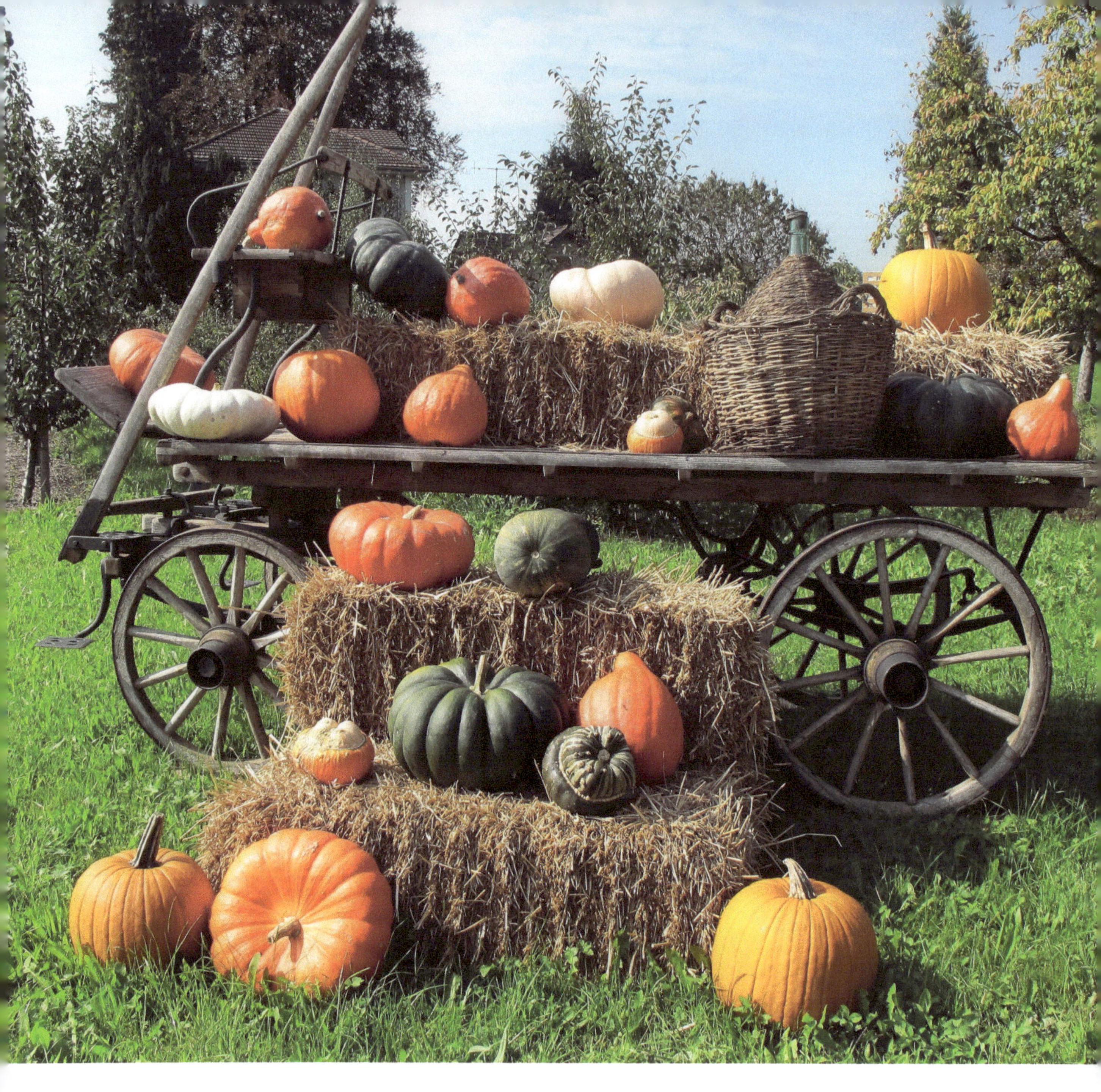

Pumpkins and squashes

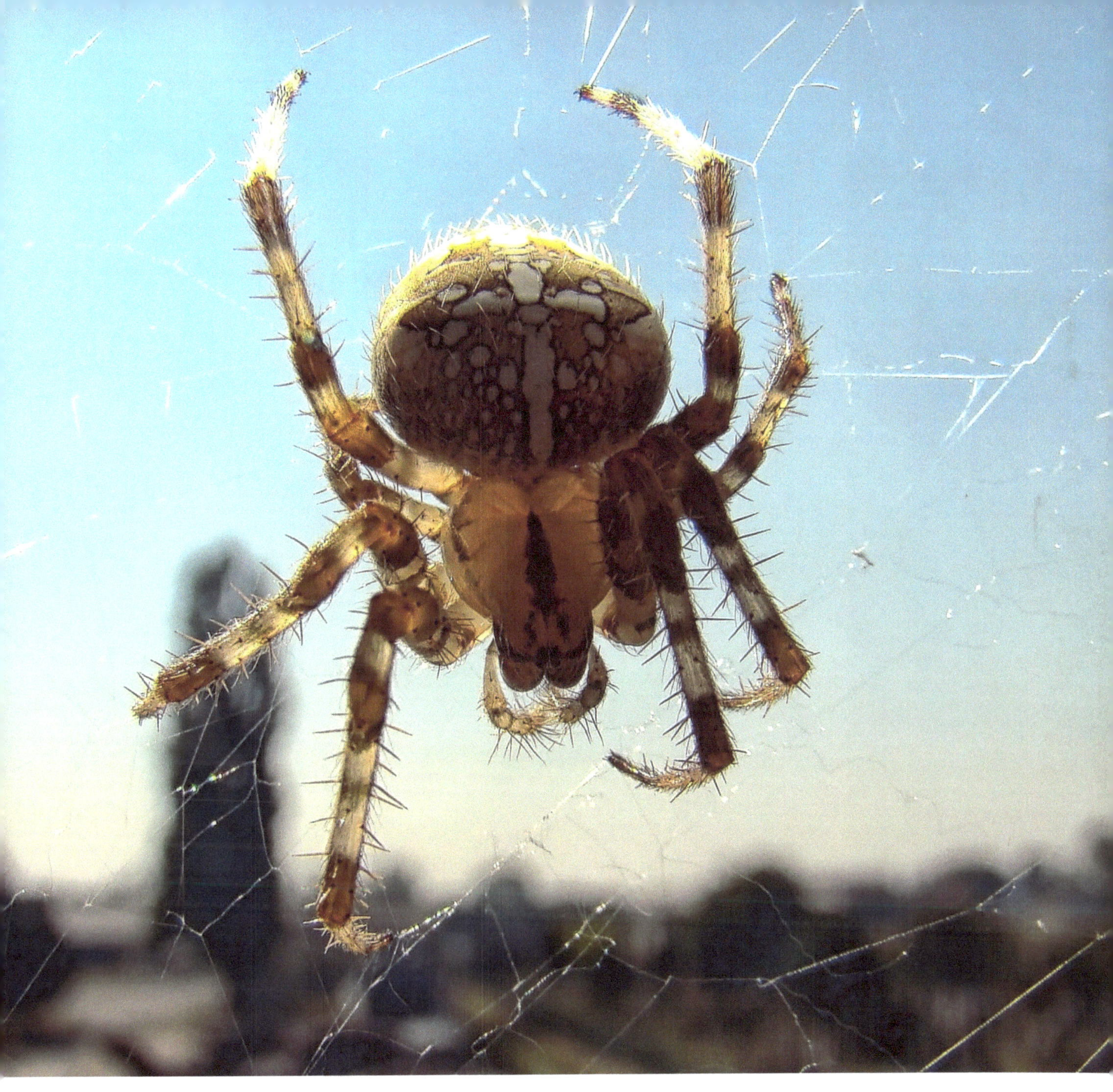

A spider

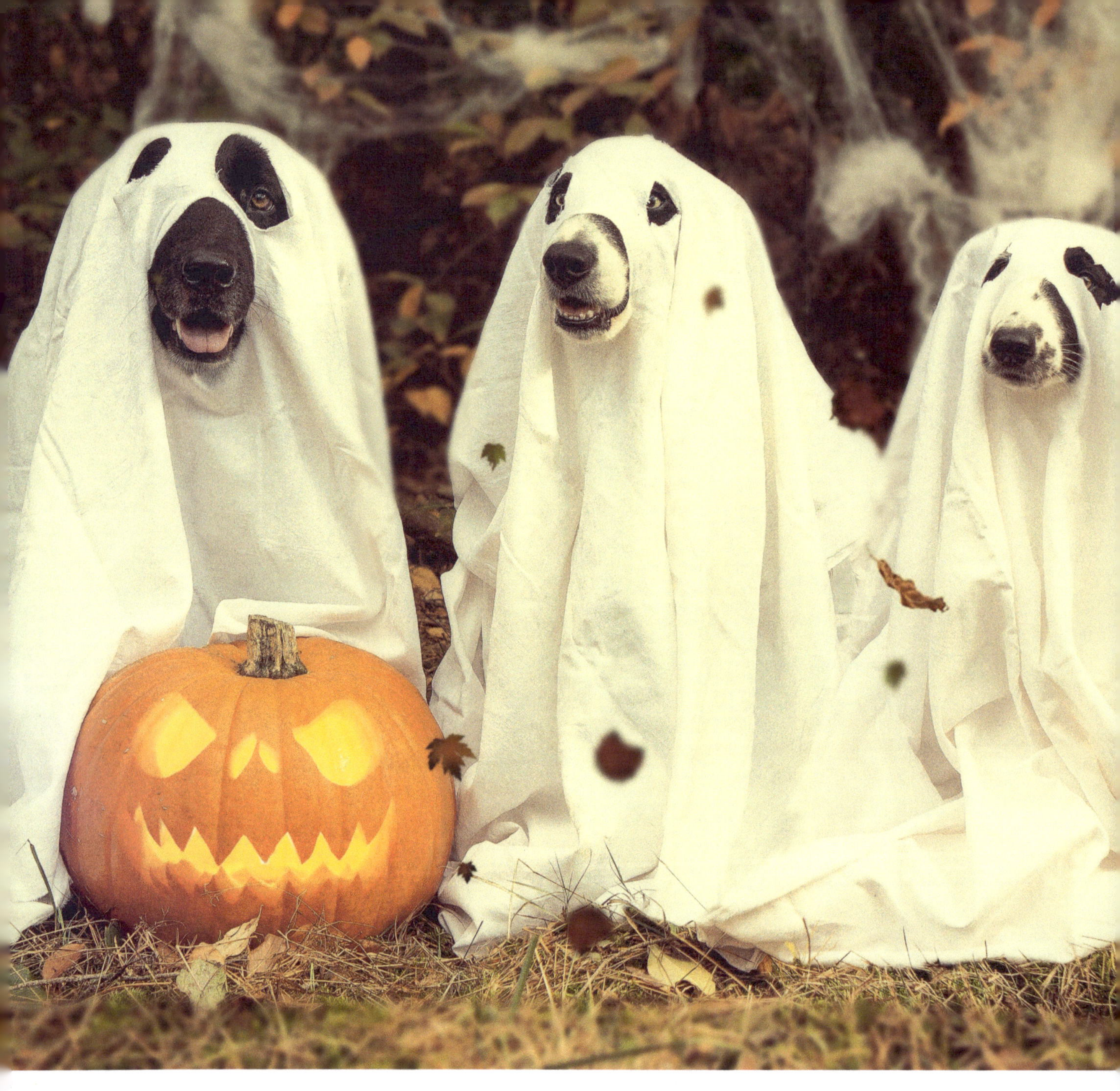

Three dogs dressed as ghosts

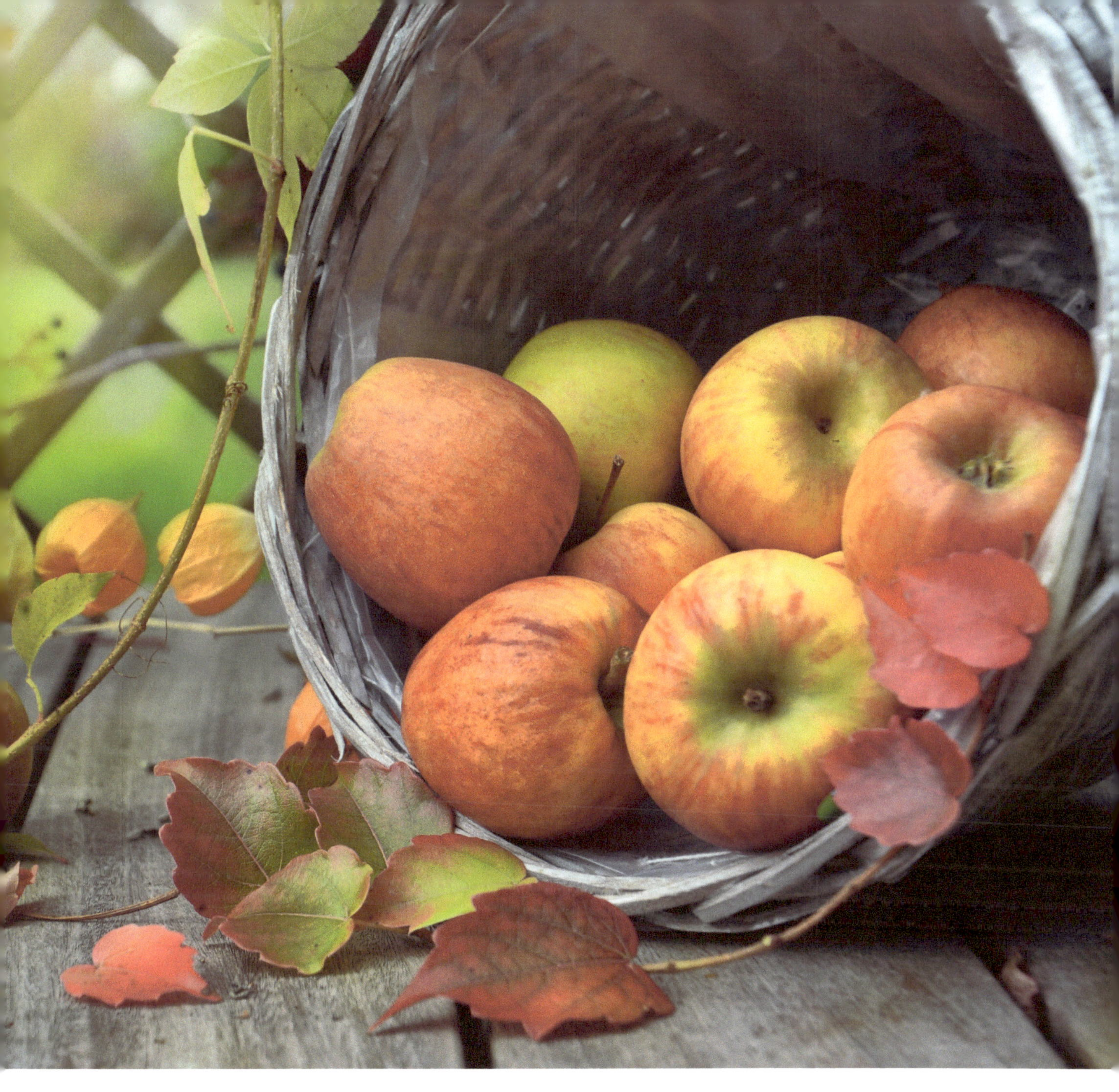

Apples

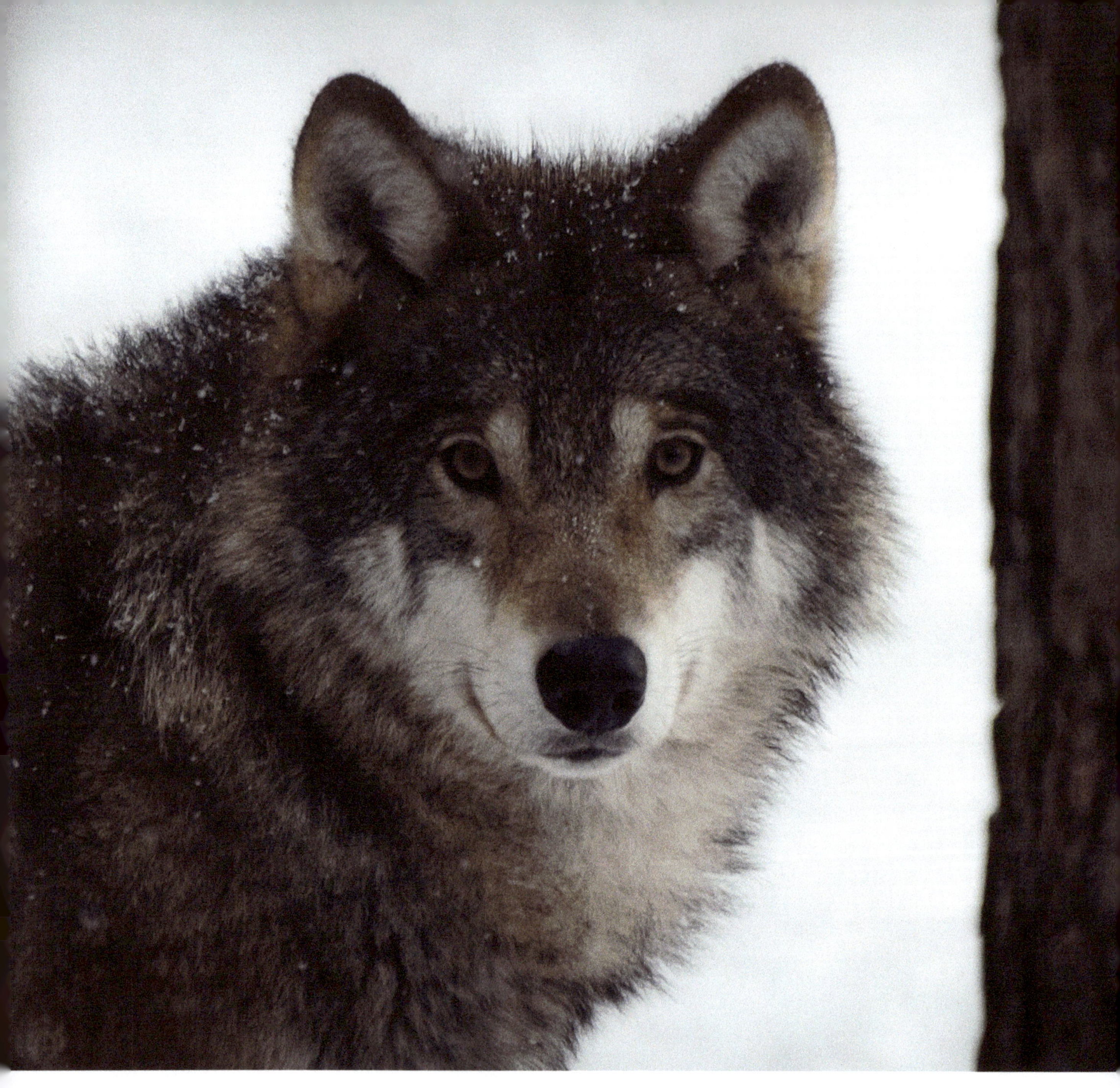

A wolf

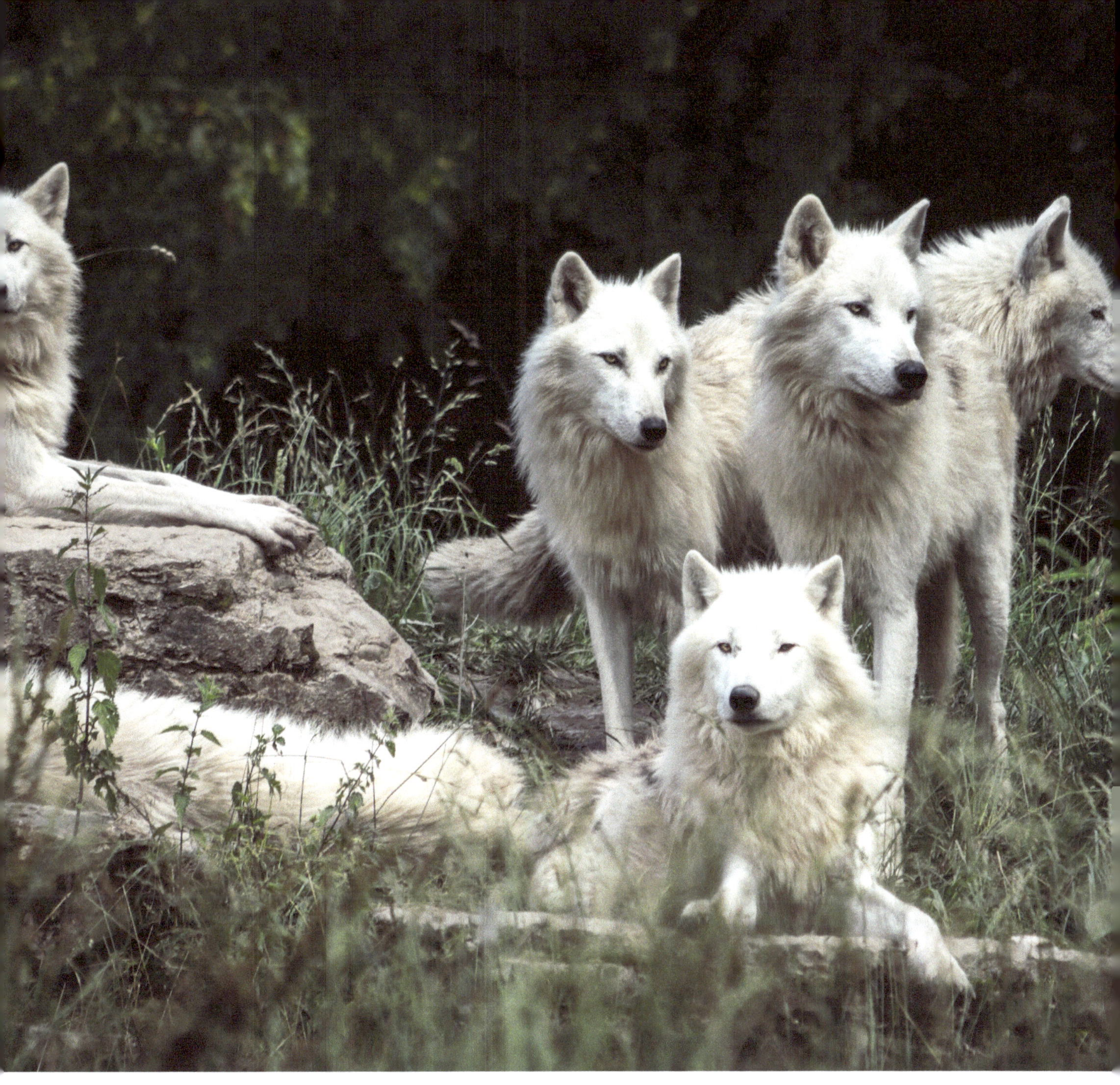

A pack of wolves

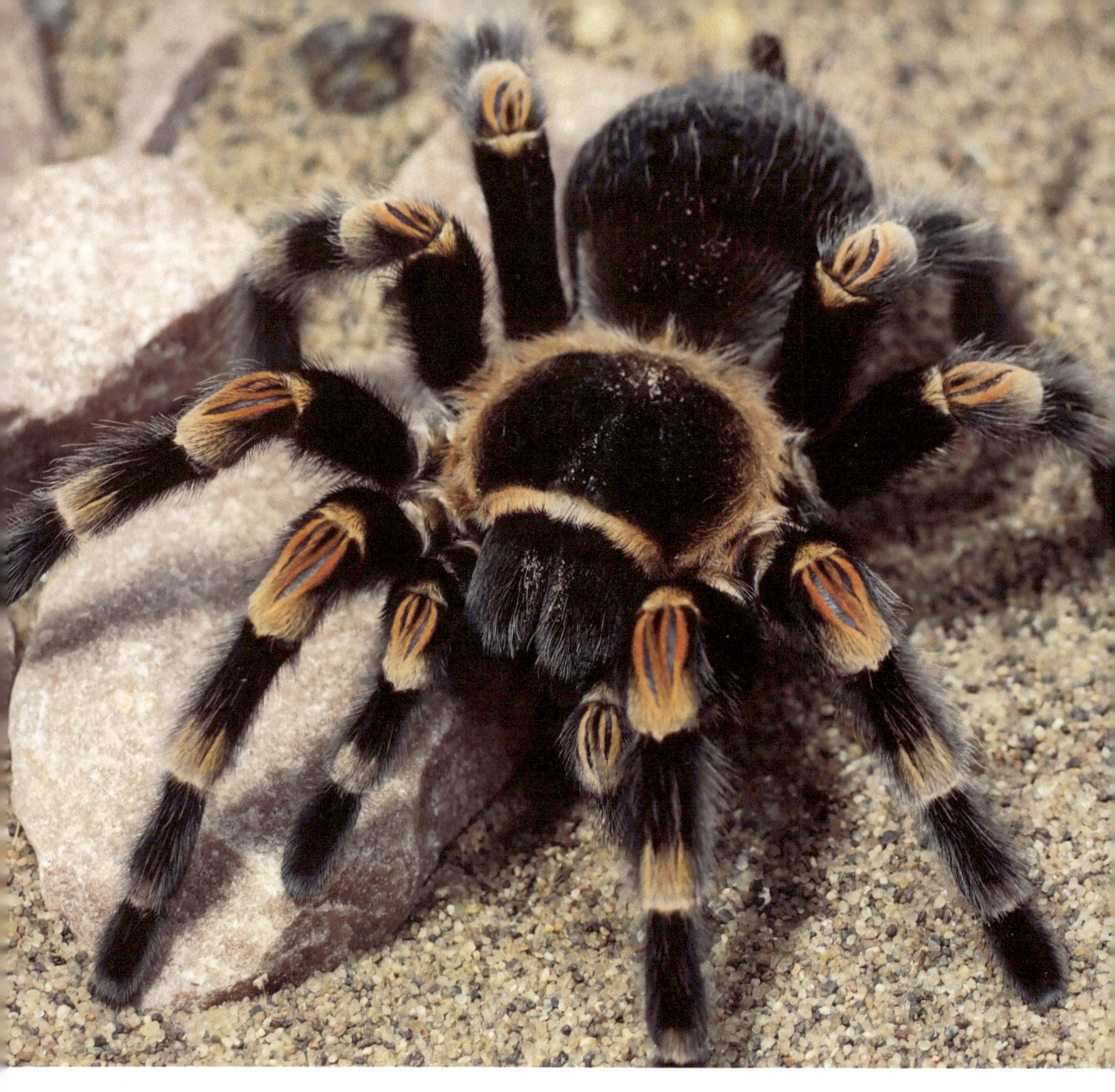

A spider

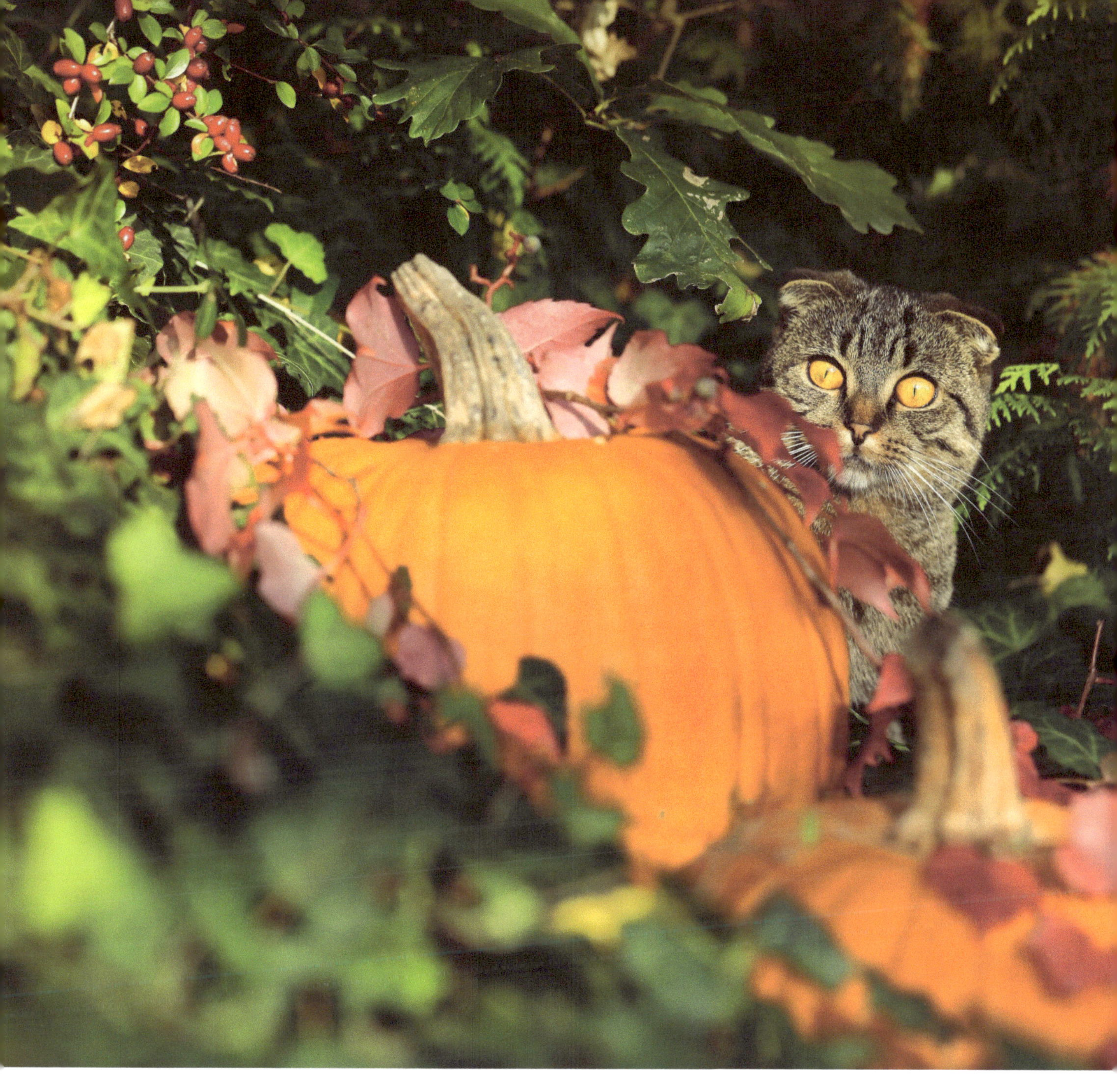

A cat behind a pumpkin

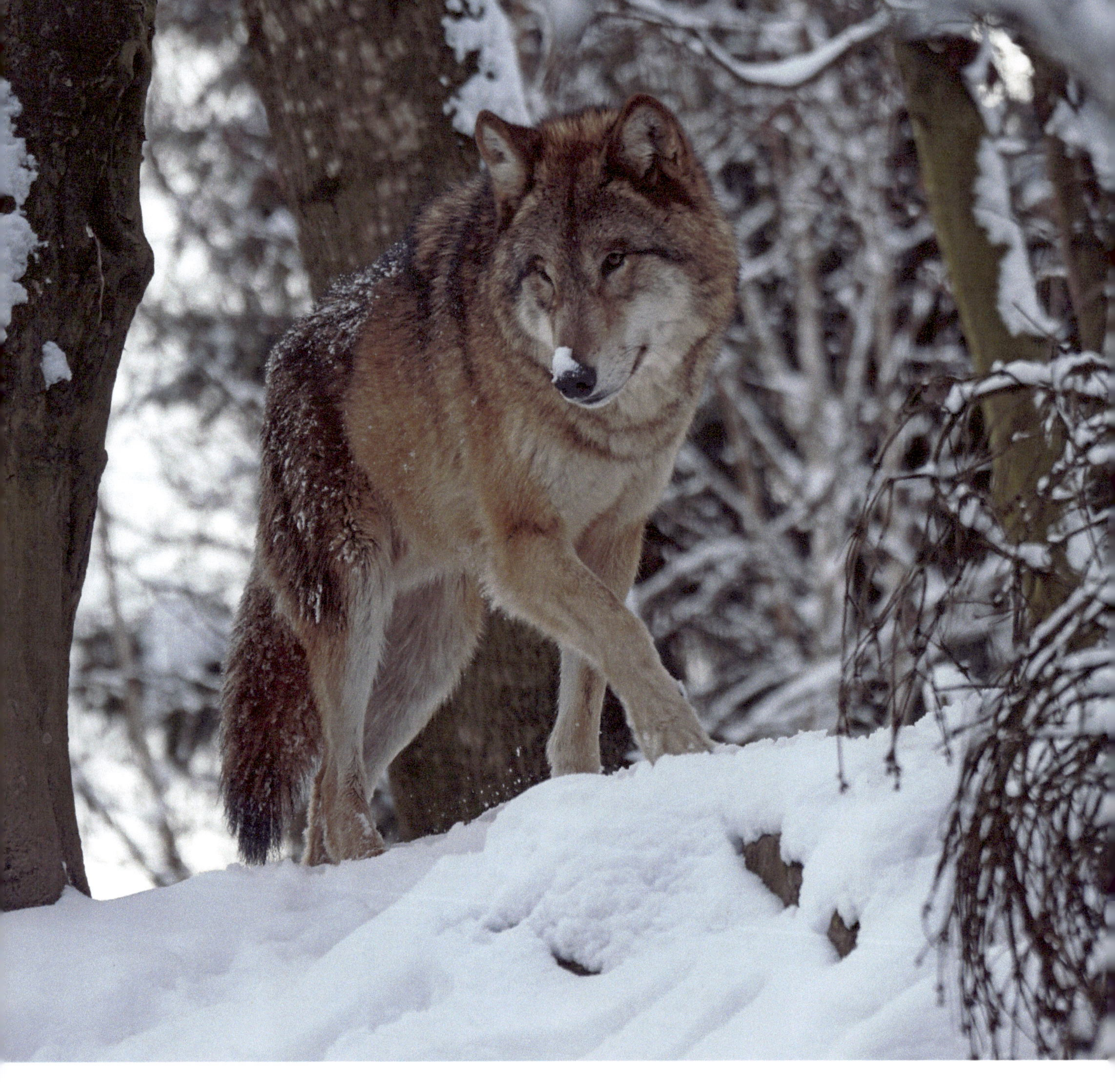

A wolf

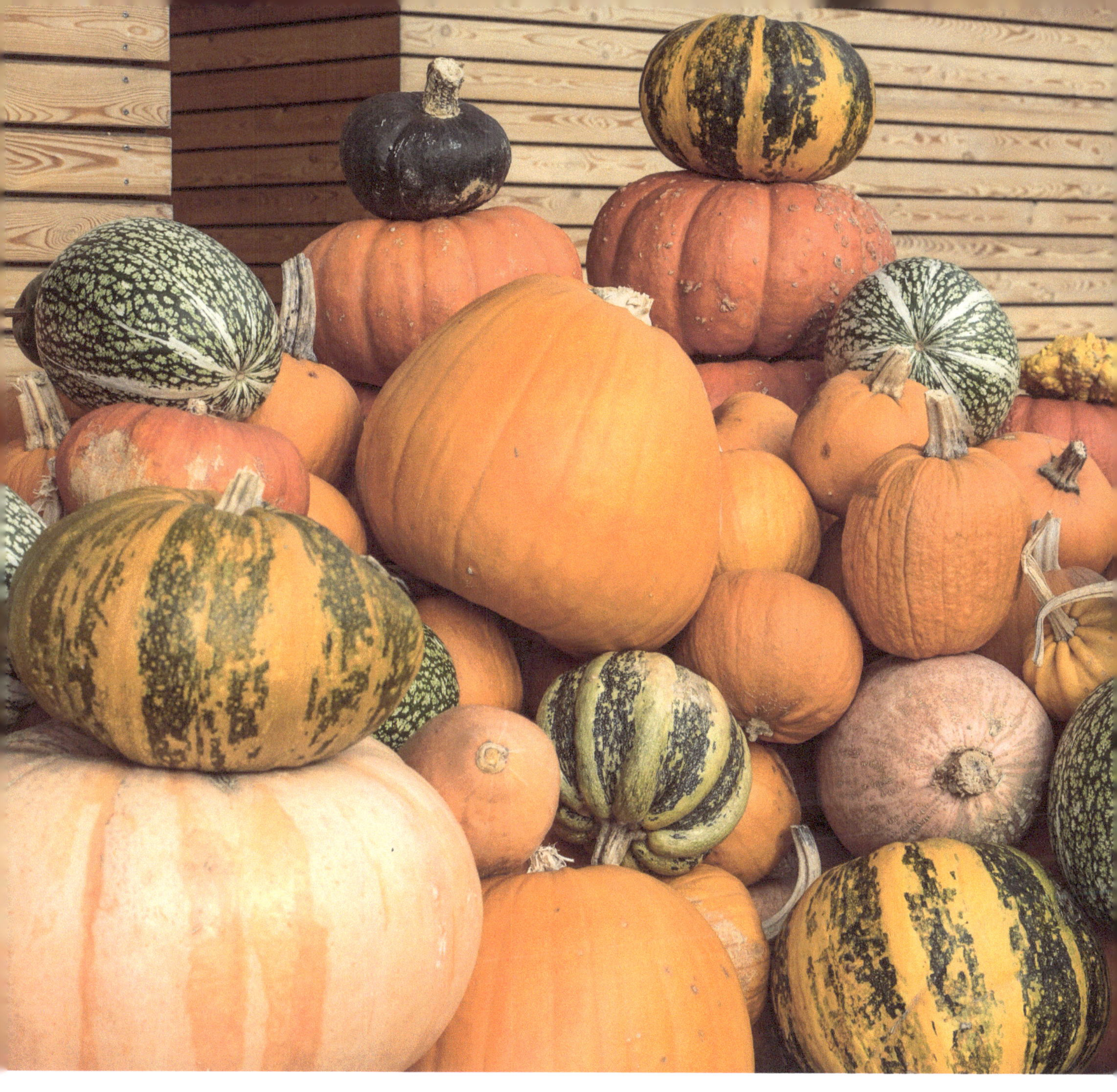

Pumpkins and squashes

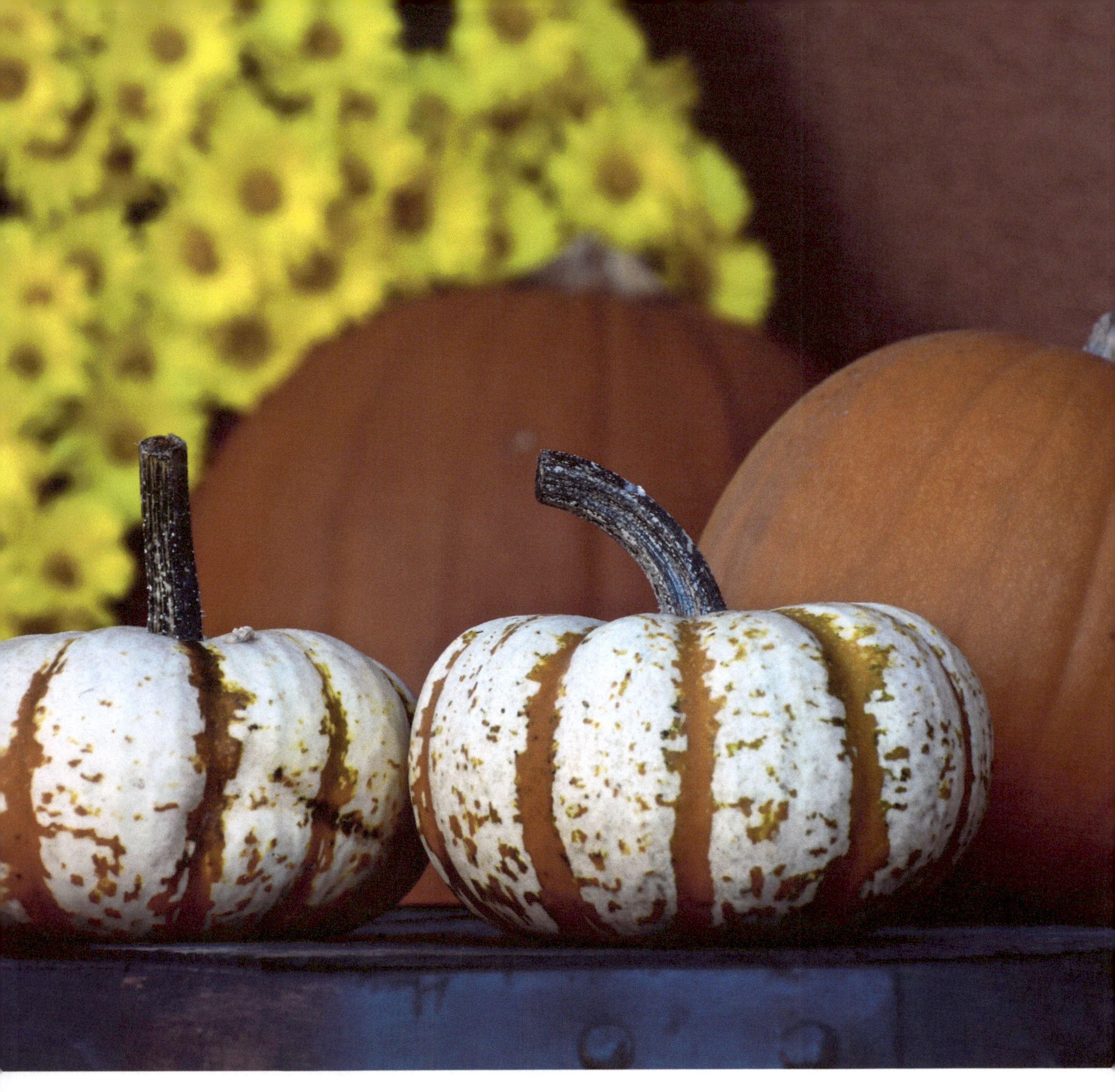

Pumpkins and squashes

www.ingramcontent.com/pod-product-compliance
Lightning Source LLC
Chambersburg PA
CBHW040152240726
48664CB00002B/672